Childbirth Without Pain

DR. PIERRE VELLAY

WITH

ALINE VELLAY, COLETTE JEANSON,
MICHELINE AND ANDRE BOURREL

Translated from the French by

DENISE LLOYD

NEW YORK
E. P. DUTTON & CO., INC.

First published in the United States, 1960
by E. P. Dutton & Co., Inc.

English translation copyright, ©, 1959, by
E. P. Dutton & Co., Inc., New York,
and George Allen & Unwin Ltd., London.

First Printing April 1960
Second Printing July 1964

Library of Congress Catalog Card Number: 60-9746

Translated from parts of the following.

Principes et pratique de l'accouchement sans douleur
Témoinages sur l'accouchement sans douleur
La méthode complète de préparation à l'accouchement sans douleur

Published in France by Editions du Seuil

Contents

Part One

BACKGROUND TO THE METHOD

Part Two

THE COMPLETE TRAINING FOR CHILDBIRTH WITHOUT PAIN

Part Three

PERSONAL ACCOUNTS OF THE METHOD

Introduction

THE search for ways to make childbirth more comfortable has occupied the attention of many men and women for a great many years. Recently this search has taken a new direction. The concept of psychosomatic unity has given this trend its impetus. The idea that mind and body are one, and that the "mind" (which includes the intellect and the emotions) can influence body function and vice versa is not new. What *is* new is the study of exactly how the mind influences the body, how the body influences the mind, and how this relationship can be favorably affected.

The conscious application of psychosomatic principles in the practice of obstetrics is a development of the past two decades. This is a fact which can be readily verified by a perusal of obstetrical textbooks which were current in 1940. One searches their pages in vain for a mention of anxiety or a discussion of the effect of the emotions on pregnancy and labor. Except for a few pioneers whose work was largely neglected, there was little interest in studying the pregnant woman as a *person* who was having a baby.

Many years ago one of the pioneers, Dr. Grantly Dick-Read, suggested that the pain in labor was the result of anxiety which, in turn, resulted from preconditioning by the mores and attitudes of modern society. His work attracted little notice until the years immediately following World War II. At that time enough interest was generated in the United States to stimulate many studies in psychosomatic obstetrics. Those who participated in these studies, both the women who had the babies and the doctors who delivered them, became convinced that through education, training, and adequate support women could enjoy a comfortable delivery.

At the same time that these principles were evolving in this country, a similar line of study was being followed in Russia. Based on the Pavlovian concept of conditioning, a system of education, training, and support was developed so that women were enabled to have their babies without pain. A French obstetrician, Dr. Fernand Lamaze, instituted this system in France.

His associate, Dr. Pierre Vellay, here describes this system and I am glad to introduce his book to the American public. Not only parents, but those who are directly and indirectly concerned with making delivery painless and pleasurable will surely welcome Dr. Vellay's contribution to the growing literature on psychosomatic obstetrics with the conviction that it will be of real help to those mothers who read it.

FREDERICK W. GOODRICH, JR., M.D.

New London, Connecticut
January, 1960

Preface

In this volume we have tried to include everything about the psychoprophylactic method of childbirth without pain that would interest a pregnant woman who knows nothing of the method. We have also tried to write concisely and in a way that will be intelligible to every reader. First we have considered the main principles and then gone on to the practical side. We have published the lectures exactly as we delivered them.

We have included a series of case-histories. They are simple, interesting from a human point of view and many-sided. Every woman reader can imagine her own case in them, and, we hope, will be encouraged to take the training.

This book is the result of much hard work by a team under the late Dr. Lamaze whom we very much miss. Assistants, midwives, doctors and mothers have all played a part at the Pierre-Rouquès trade-union centre, where the method has been evolved. We are deeply grateful to all who helped us.

We hope that this book will make each woman reader anxious to experience the indescribable joy of childbirth without pain.

P.V.
A.V.

Foreword

THIS book is dedicated to all future mothers and to all women who have already had the experience of childbirth without pain. We hope that it will give confidence to the mothers of the future, and that its detailed information, with the evidence of other women like themselves, will create a feeling of security in one of the most important events of their lives.

The book is written in gratitude to the women who have tried our method. They completely changed our ideas on the subject, and by their courage they liberated the sex in general from its burdensome and degrading past. There is still a long way to go. Women must teach their daughters—early in puberty, so that they can go through all the important stages of life without difficulty.

We are not entering into the scientific basis of the method or how it has been put into practice. What we do here is to gather impressions written by women about childbirth. Their accounts are faithful, instructive and sometimes moving. We have supervised so many childbirths without pain that we cannot publish all the reports. We have had to select—not an easy task.

As we have read these accounts, which cover nearly four years, we have noticed considerable development both in content and style. At the beginning the women's accounts were cold clinical records—though full of information for us. For the first time in medicine, the subject of an experiment was describing her sensations. The accounts were like miniature police reports. But quite quickly the impersonal tone changed. The women began to express their feelings and thoughts.

C.W.P. seems to release psychological tensions and so to be curative from the psychological point of view. The woman studies herself, discovers her problems and finds a solution. C.W.P. goes beyond pure obstetrics. It is women's victory, and it transforms their position in the family and society.

9

In selecting the women's accounts, we have tried to help readers to recognize themselves and discover their own problems. But it is a large subject, and the book is not as full as we should like. Also, our experience, though considerable, is still incomplete. We have not yet discovered the full range of human reactions. Only by continuing to work together shall we be able gradually to explore the vast territory before us.

Our task needs patience, but it is exciting. We want to discover the mechanisms and influences—internal and external—which make the human machine work well or badly.

In this age, with its radio, television, newspapers and cinema, a matter concerning millions of women was bound to be widely publicized. Discoveries in all fields of science should be published as soon as possible to give people the opportunity of benefiting. Medicine cannot remain outside modern forms of communication. It would risk stagnation. Any means of relieving human suffering must be made known as soon as possible.

Childbirth without pain is a new phenomenon. It could not be kept among a few initiates. It belongs to all women, and women have helped to spread the information. Childbirth without pain depends on education. Our first task was to make the method known; then to educate the women who might benefit, and finally to educate all women.

This book, therefore, is part of the education of the public.

P.V.
A.V.

PART ONE

BACKGROUND TO THE METHOD

I

Dr. Lamaze: a biographical Note

DOCTORS send us letters from all over the world, reporting on their experiences. In the last few months the patients they are training have repeatedly asked, 'Who is Dr. Lamaze?' Here is an answer.

Spring, 1947. He walked slowly and heavily, limping a little because of a war-wound. He was strongly built and wore no hat in all weathers. But he did carry an umbrella to protect his book as well as himself. When I (Dr. Vellay) first saw him in the doorway of a nursing home, he looked like a statue. He had a black beard, which he afterwards shaved, and a high, broad, domed forehead out of proportion to his small aquiline nose. His eyes were bright and brimming over with kindness, but they also could express serious thought and feelings. The whole of his imposing person radiated good nature and sympathy, and everyone liked him. The staff of the hospital spoke well of him; indeed one never heard an evil word of him. He knew all the obstetricians, and they all seemed to think highly of him. I often saw him—going from Porte de Saint-Cloud tube station to the hospital, with his regular step, head bowed and eyes fixed on his book, which he carried wrapped in his morning paper.

He was indifferent to his surroundings, not noticing the crowd and passing through it like an automaton. One day he boarded the tube at Porte de Saint-Cloud and sat down next to one of his friends. The friend did not speak because Dr. Lamaze was reading. The doctor got out at Sèvres-Babylone, still engrossed in his book, without noticing that his friend was there.

He was overwhelmed with work, but he never seemed in a hurry. He generally travelled by bus or tube, as then he had a chance to read and he could be punctual. He was as punctual as a clock.

He loved books, and treated them with respect, cutting the pages carefully. He could not bear to see them dog-eared. His whole life seemed a quest for knowledge.

At that time I had not heard his voice, but I wanted to.

Autumn, 1947. One day I went to see him to discuss possible collaboration in his work. I had the feeling that we resembled one another both in our activities and our minds. I went to his dark flat, and was struck by its simplicity. The door opened. Lamaze was there with a smile lighting up his face. A great human warmth emanated from him. He held out his strong hand saying, 'Good morning, my dear Vellay. Very pleased to meet you.'

He fascinated me, and at first I did not notice his study, which was small and dark. It looked more like the study of a literary man than of a doctor. Only two seats were empty. I sat down opposite to Lamaze, and then noticed that desk, table, mantelpiece, bookcases—even the floor—were covered with books.

Timidly I gave him a summary of my career. We exchanged ideas, and found we had many in common—a firm basis for collaboration. His deep voice, which was sometimes difficult to understand, gave me confidence and—like his presence—a sense of goodwill. As I left I knew that there was a strong bond between us and that nothing could change our new friendship.

How could this solitary dreamer suddenly leave his world of books and throw himself into controversy? He did not seem made for conflict. For thirty years he had divided his time between work and the acquisition of knowledge. He was also a gourmet; he knew the best wines as he knew historical dates or the biographies of famous men.

He was in turn 'soldier, rebel and citizen' in the word of Yves Farge. It was the two world wars that made him break with a life that had been up to then sufficient for his needs. During the war he became friendly through his profession with P. Rouquès. When the maternity home at the metal workers' polyclinic was opened, Rouquès asked Lamaze to direct it. It was then that I visited Lamaze in his study and we began our collaboration. For four years we worked side by side developing the clinic. Our study of childbirth without pain strengthened our unity.

The workers' home developed very quickly. 'I don't know how to give orders. I trust everyone, but I can't bear to see my confidence betrayed.' This attitude of Lamaze's was to be still more valuable during the experiments with C.W.P. And we have repaid his confidence. We have created a unified team in which everyone has his place and rôle.

In September, 1950, the World Congress of Gynaecology attracted the most eminent specialists to Paris. Professor Nicolaiev of Leningrad took advantage of his visit and went to see the Rouquès maternity home. He talked modestly of his own attempt to make childbirth painless by the psychoprophylactic method. His information had its effect. Rouquès asked Lamaze to join the medical delegation which was to go to Russia in September, 1951. Then a shadow fell. Rouquès was seriously ill and unable to go, and his death prevented his hearing of the remarkable contact with the Russians that his delegation achieved. Lamaze had consented to visit Russia and interrupt his work for the first time. The trip completely changed his life.

When he set out he had a secret purpose. He wanted to discover if Russian women really gave birth without pain—as Professor Nicolaiev had asserted. The fact seemed wonderful and incredible. Lamaze's own long experience seemed to prove that only drugs could deaden the pain of childbirth.

The French delegation had a full programme in Russia, but Lamaze held to his purpose. He wanted to see a woman give birth without pain. The days passed. Visits to hospitals followed visits to institutes. Lamaze saw and talked to women who had given birth without pain. The method was explained to him. As the time for his departure approached, he became more and more anxious to see the event. He pestered the interpreters and the authorities, and declared that he would not report on this method when he returned unless absolute proof were given him.

On 4 September, 1951, he was visiting the Pavlov Institute at Koltouchi when he was summoned to see a birth in Professor Nicolaiev's department at Leningrad. For six hours Lamaze remained at the woman's bedside, vigilant and yet profoundly affected. He watched the progress of labour and the woman's reactions. He saw how she was relaxed both in expression and body. Guided by the doctor, she brought her child into the world without pain, with complete simplicity and the most perfect confidence.

The scene seemed beautiful to Lamaze. He was in a state of great excitement when he met the members of the delegation. Dr. Moutier describes how he seemed rejuvenated. He was full of enthusiasm like the scientist who sees the end of his research. During the evening he could talk of nothing else. 'That woman,' he said, 'will always remain in my memory like a source of light.' From then on he had one aim only—to give Frenchwomen the same experience.

I myself shall never forget his voice, full of warmth and enthusiasm, when he told us, on his return, of the experience. He described it in minute detail. For him it surpassed all the other events of the trip. To us the event was surprising, even incredible. It took all our confidence in Lamaze to make us believe it. But we knew him to be thoughtful and level-headed, and finally we were convinced—and stimulated by his enthusiasm. We wanted to try the experiment ourselves and assess it.

We decided to set to work at once. At the start the literature and equipment available were very limited, but the general goodwill and the women's confidence and understanding soon brought us undeniable proof of painless childbirth. Thanks to Pavlov's research on conditional reflexes, which had been adapted to obstetrics by such doctors as Velvolski and Nicolaiev, Russian women, we now knew, were giving birth without pain, and their experience could be passed on to other women.

Lamaze's success surprised even himself. He paid a second visit to Russia in February, 1955, and talked to Professor Lionid Stipanov, director of the Institute of Gynaecology and Obstetrics at Moscow. He was told that nearly forty delegations like his own had come from the East and West. They, too, had seen demonstrations. But he was the only one who had tried to apply the method when he returned to his own country. His Russian colleague esteemed him for this. So did we, his followers. Humanist and doctor as he was, he showed that science has no frontiers. He might have said like Pasteur: 'I ask neither your political nor religious views, but what is your suffering?'

Tirelessly, persistently, Lamaze continued, overcoming obstacles daily and relying more and more on us whom he had convinced. He ignored fatigue, and worked ceaselessly at the task he had set himself, certain, as he said, that truth is always triumphant. And the truth was not confined to France. He made it shine out from the small maternity home attached to the Rouquès centre like a ray of hope for all women.

From all countries doctors poured in, always curious and sometimes sceptical. After repeated demonstrations they left convinced, stimulated and anxious to apply the discovery. This success, which adds prestige to French medicine, was, in the last resort, due to the women who submitted themselves for experiment. At the beginning Lamaze would say repeatedly, 'Let's keep on working and demonstrate the truth every day of childbirth without pain. Women will know how to use the discovery.'

And now an important event in French social history has taken place. Women of all origins and religions, all colours and classes, realize that their position has changed. We no longer believe that the human being is an animal.

The late Pope, in his speech of 8 February, 1956, recognized the value of the psychoprophylactic method. The prospect of more humanistic medicine may now open up. Everyone will gain something. As a foreign doctor said, 'In twenty years' time the new generation of women will remember Lamaze with gratitude. He fundamentally changed childbirth and the very condition of women in the Western world.'

2

Historical

THE first experiments in childbirth without pain were based on hypnosis—which was also used with some success for surgical anaesthesia. Between 1880 and 1890 many attempts were made, and many of these were partially successful. Quite often women who benefited were special cases—victims of hysteria, for example. In 1890, however, le Menant des Chesnais, Luys, Panton and then Auvard obtained excellent results from normal people. But hypnosis could be used only by specialists and only to a limited extent. On the other hand, as Dr. Henri Vermorel notes, these doctors' experience 'is the first illustration of the reality of childbirth without pain.'[1]

Later much research went on to improve the method. Joire, in 1889, used suggestion when the patient was awake, but he, too, could not try it on a large scale.

Meanwhile hypnotic experiments were being made abroad, in Germany, Belgium, England and Austria. But it was in Russia that the method developed most; and in 1902 twenty out of twenty-eight women who had been hypnotized gave birth without pain. But the method was empiric. It was then that Pavlov's work provided a scientific basis for hypnosis; he explained its psychological mechanism and so opened new doors to research.

From 1920 onwards Platonov applied this technique to childbirth. With Velvoski he had studied suggestion and hypnosis in surgery, obstetrics, gynaecology and stomatology. Nicolaiev and he attempted to go further. They allowed women to give birth in a waking state under post-hypnotic influence. Between 1922 and 1938 much work was done on suggestion and hypnosis. Training was begun. The work

[1] *L'accouchement sans douleur par la méthode psychoprophylactique à la lunière de l'enseignement psychologique de Pavlov*. Camugli, Ed., Lyon.

was very successful. Vigdorovitch obtained 80 per cent success from 4,000 childbirths in the waking or half-waking state.

Finally in 1938 Skrobanski, stressing the importance of suggestion, maintained that it must be used in prenatal clinics, independently of the suggestion used during confinement. 'The woman who has been prepared for analgesia and who has confidence,' he writes, 'submits easily to any method, while the woman who is convinced that freedom from pains is impossible will feel pain with any method.'

Meanwhile, Nicolaiev writes: 'The analgesic technique in obstetrics must be applied to a large number of people. . . . The doctor must reshape the mind of the woman who has been brought up with the idea that pain is inevitable and unalterable.'[1]

At about this time Dr. Dick Read in England discovered the psychological character of pain and hence the value of training. But in 1945, in spite of all experiments, hypno-suggestion, as Velvoski emphasized, was not generally applied. In nearly thirty years, only eight thousand childbirths without pain had taken place. But they served as a foundation for the next step—psychoprophylaxis as the chief means of removing the pains of childbirth.

In 1949 Nicolaiev and Platanov supported Velvoski's ideas at a Karkov conference. The work of the Pavlov school had given them a scientific foundation. Nicolaiev declared that the pain of childbirth—its manifestation, character and strength—depended on the nervous system and the relationship between cortex and sub-cortex. He proposed the term psychoprophylaxis.

The next year, in June, 1950, at a session of the Academy of Sciences, the physiological and therapeutic value of the spoken word was emphasized. In 1951 the Academy of Medicine and the Ministry of Public Health organized a conference at which Velvoski, Pavlov, Nicolaiev and their colleagues described the new method. They had perfected it little by little, and now used it in Karkov, Moscow and Leningrad. Their results were conclusive.

In July, 1951, the Russian Government ordered that the method should be applied to the whole country. In that year Dr. Lamaze returned from Russia and introduced the psychoprophylactic method into France. The French were the second nation in the world to use it, China coming in just after. At the beginning Dr. Lamaze and his assistants had very little scientific literature. They used the notes they

[1] cf. Dr. Henri Vermorel, op. cit.

had brought back from Russia, and they asked the women themselves to write reports on their experiences.

The various experiments were gradually linked—to the general advantage. The French method, which had originated in Russia, added innovations which in turn were valuable to the Russians. Then the French method spread—to forty-four countries in the last two years. The work of other countries, published later, strengthens the French experiment, which again is reacting on Russia and China.

3

General Survey

PSYCHOPROPHYLAXIS is verbal analgesia based on the training of the pregnant woman. It is quite different from other methods of obstetrical analgesia. It depends on words as therapeutic agents (Pavlov's second system). Its basis is the use of conditional reflexes, studied by Pavlov and his pupils and applied to obstetrics by Russian doctors such as Velvoski and Nicolaiev.

It attempts to equilibrate the brain (cortex) of the pregnant woman by creating during pregnancy complex chains of conditioned reflexes which will be applicable at the confinement. The pregnant woman learns to give birth as the child learns to read or swim. She completes this education, and so understands the simple mechanism of childbirth and can adapt herself when her confinement arrives. She gets rid of the bad influences and memories she has previously accumulated, which may inhibit her in the act of birth.

Women lose the passive attitude which most of them adopt when facing childbirth. They know what is going to happen and learn to adapt themselves and control the changes which occur in their bodies during labour. Like expert engineers with perfect machines they control, direct and regulate their bodies.

For a long time doctors have been relieving childbirth pain by anaesthesia. Chloroform first and then the most varied drugs have been used—according to the development of biochemistry and pharmacology. There have been four possible modes of attack:

1. To reduce local sensation in the uterus.

2. To interrupt the relaying of painful sensations between the uterus and the brain. (Epidural or continuous caudal block, infiltration of gangli or nerves from the uterus.)

21

3. To diminish or suppress the consciousness of pain (scopolamine, etc.).

4. To act on the three local factors of transmission of sensation by partly or completely anaesthetizing the woman (modern closed-circuit analgesia).

All these methods were interesting and useful, and they have stood the test of time. But the use of drugs is not without dangers for both mother and child. A method was needed which would incorporate two basic principles:

A. Non-toxicity for mother and child.

B. Active and complete participation of the woman, who is carrying out one of the most important acts of her life.

In all normal cases the psychoprophylactic method fulfils these two conditions perfectly.

The method is not a trick as some people think. There is no ready-made formula. The method has its rules and disciplines, and it must be applied conscientiously and intelligently. It is not an easy method for woman, assistant or doctor. It needs co-operative effort, but that effort enriches all taking part. It results in 'giving of life in the best conditions for the mother as well as for the child.'

Pavlov, who studied the salivary secretion—the so-called 'psychical secretion'—in the dog, introduced the idea of the reflex as a basic factor in human physiology. He showed that this reflex is an active response allowing the animal to adapt itself to its changing environment. The reflex is neither an elementary nor simple phenomenon. It depends on the activity of nervous processes such as excitation or inhibition, and it corresponds to varied and complex reactions.

Pavlov described two types of reflex:

A. Absolute reflexes, such as the defence reflex, or the salivary reflex. They are inherited. Their nervous centre is subcortical, mesen-cephalon, bulb or spinal cord. They ensure the first reactions of the human being to the outside world, but they cannot maintain an equilibrium between the individual, who varies continuously, and the environment in which he lives.

B. Acquired, temporary reflexes. They depend on the effect of environment, and form the conditioned reflexes. The best known is the salivary reflexes. When food accompanied by the sound of a bell is given to a dog, the sound alone will presently make it salivate.

In the cerebral cortex two centres of excitation have arisen—one caused by the sound of the bell and the other by the tasting of food. Between these two points a new pathway is temporarily established.

'The world in which we live is not chaotic. It is not made up of a casual accumulation of things. Objective laws rule it. Stimuli do not act on the body in an unordered way. In their immense variety one can see series of signals which are repeated in a comparatively orderly manner.

To a group of given signals a functional structure (a stereotype) which can act on its own to a certain extent ('a dynamic stereotype') responds within the nervous system.'[1]

Simple or complex conditioned reflexes are not independent. They help to create nervous functional structures to which Pavlov has given the name of 'dynamic stereotypes'. These are sorts of 'formulae' of conditioning, different from the sum of simple connexions. The formula holds as long as all the stimuli continue—even if they are reversed —but is destroyed if an unusual stimulus is introduced. Very different formulae, more or less complicated, can be created.

'During confinement it is not so much the isolated small stimuli that have an effect but the signals grouped in dynamic stereotypes.'[2]

The dynamic stereotype is the physiological basis of human beings' activities. The various more or less complicated formulae correspond to the multiple situations of our daily lives. We deal with them in this way, and so constantly adapt ourselves to our environment.

Yet there are limits to the organization of such stereotypes. Our nervous system must select the stimuli it receives. Otherwise there would be anarchy, and we could not follow any continued activity. Selection takes place through equilibrium between two fundamental nervous processes—positive excitation and negative excitation (inhibition or braking).

'In the process of equilibration between the body and the outside world, the two processes intervene, one of excitation and one of inhibition.' (Pavlov)

Any positive excitation in the cortex tends to be diffused, but this diffusion induces the opposite process—inhibition. A struggle begins between the positive activity (excitation) and the negative activity. It ends in a concentration and selection in the centres of activity

[1] *L'Accounchement sans douleur par la méthode psychoprophylactique à la lumière de l'enseignement physiologique de Pavlov.* Henri Vermorel.
[2] Idem.

eliminating any other secondary activity. Negative activity can be conditioned as well as positive activity. From a stimulus an inhibiting conditioned stimulus can be created.

Let us take an example. On a dog's leg are placed five small devices to stimulate the skin—D, C, B, A, Z, (from top to bottom). Apparatus z makes an inhibiting stimulus of the secretion. Remember that the topographical relations of the apparatus are reproduced in the cerebral cortex. Apparatus z is switched on. An inhibiting wave immediately develops, and for thirty seconds stimulation by apparatus A, B, C, D, produces nothing. It is inhibited by the cerebral cortex. After a minute, apparatus A (the nearest to z) is still producing no secretion, but apparatus B, farther away, produces one drop, C, still farther, three drops, and D, farther still, five drops. Two minutes later we get two drops from A, five from B, eight from C, and ten from D. After another four minutes we get four drops from A, and ten from each of B, C, and D. Finally, six minutes later, we get the full effect from each of A, B, C, and D—say ten drops each. Inhibition is limited to point z. This experiment of Krasnogorski's shows, very exactly, how excitation and inhibition work together.

The whole of Pavlov's work consists of equally exact and careful

KRASNOGORSKI'S EXPERIMENT

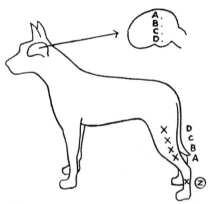

If the point Z is stimulated: Inhibition 'braking'

Time:	0	1'	2'	4'	6'
D	0	5	10	10	10
C	0	3	8	10	10
B	0	1	5	10	10
A	0	0	2	4	10

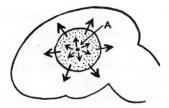

I. → *Positive excitation and its spread.*

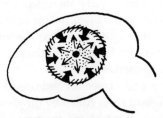

II. ➡ *Inhibition induced.*

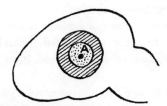

III. *'Braking'—concentration of activity.*

Theoretical diagrams explaining the phenomena of excitation, inhibition and 'braking'.

experiments. From these emerges the possibility of a relationship between the woman's active participation in childbirth and the inhibition of stimuli coming from her uterus—the elimination of the pain.

Two types of stimuli reach the cortex: (a) Those coming from the outside world and transmitted by the sense organs, comprising exteroception. (b) Those coming from our viscera and comprising interoception.

Pavlov showed the unity of these two systems, and that their equilibrium is a condition of existence.

In the dynamic stereotypes there is a close association of internal and external signals. A special form of signalling exists in man—

language. Pavlov has called it the second system of signalling. Words by their meaning enable the human being to have precise and complex dynamic stereotypes, far superior to those formed by the animal through direct signals. To adapt a woman to childbirth there cannot be a better instrument than language.

Before childbirth without pain the untrained woman was under the influence of three unfavourable factors.

1. Her exhaustion was greatly increased by emotions and fears caused by her ignorance and that of people round her, by gossip and bogus scientific publications. She was incapable of acting purposefully in her confinement and could not inhibit the stimuli coming from the uterus (uterine interoceptors).

2. Bad upbringing had caused a conditioned connexion between confinement and imagined pain. Aided by the atmosphere in which the confinement took place, she replaced the word 'labour' by the word 'pain'. When we began our work, women found it difficult to use the word 'contraction' instead of 'pain'. After C.W.P. one said, 'It didn't hurt me from the first pain to the last'.

3. Complete cortical disorganization resulted from absence of appropriate dynamic stereotypes. This, with the lack of active participation, hindered the creation of adequate inhibition.

If the woman is to achieve well controlled activity she must be trained. Negative emotions must be suppressed and she must be shown that childbirth is a physiological natural act. Strongly positive emotions must be created. She must be shown all the enrichment that childhood brings to a woman. Absolute confidence must also be created.

Women must learn childbirth like reading and writing. They must realize the value of their conscious active participation in childbirth. They must realize the part they have to play during labour. They will be shown that childbirth is a process which they themselves can follow, control and direct. Finally, with practical training, they will by themselves create a defence mechanism and adapt their bodies to labour.

The principles of training hang together, and for success they must be treated as a unity. The teacher himself must be familiar with the higher nervous activity. He must use simple and vivid language.

Training for childbirth without pain is done in nine lectures. The first takes place in about the fourth month of pregnancy. It explains what can be gained from knowledge, and puts the woman on her guard against dangers caused by ignorance. She is taught about her body, her reproductive organs, the formation and development of the egg, the life of the foetus and the uterine cavity.

The eight other lectures are given in the last two months of pregnancy. Six of them deal with neuro-muscular training and exercises; and the seventh with uterine action during labour (dilatation of the cervix, delivery of the baby). The eighth gives an outline idea of brain mechanisms.

Then comes a film, going over the same ground with illustrations. It shows what women can do if they put the lessons into practice.

The method will have to be used nationally if it is to have the maximum effect. We shall not get the result we want until the whole population has been instructed through the public services without prejudice or opposition. In China, for example, women, public authorities and the medical profession have all worked together and provided optimum conditions.

In France results vary. This is because the method is not always used in the right way. Most of the failures are due, not to the training itself, but to its incompleteness. Doctors do not know enough. Women must insist on being trained in the proper way. Any deception or fake can only harm the woman when she is confined.

In obstetrics, as in surgery, each doctor may have his own technique. But a definite scientific method is a unity. It cannot be modified without damage. C.W.P. has suffered from being distorted. It has been given different names—natural childbirth, childbirth without fear, psychosomatic childbirth. These conceptions are valuable, and useful training is given. But the term 'childbirth without pain' is valuable in itself, as those who have studied the rôle of language agree. If the words 'without pain' are omitted, their use in obstetrical analgesia is lost. As the method develops and is better understood, the numbers of women giving birth without pain will increase.

We ourselves accept only results obtained when the method has been correctly applied—and the right disciplines submitted to. Our method makes use of words alone as an analgesic, but adds a simple rational training where physical factors play a minor part. We cannot consider results produced by another method in which gymnastics are the main factor and training counts for less—the method of Dr. Dick Read. In childbirth without pain anaesthetizing a woman is out of the question when the childbirth is normal—as it generally is. If we used anaesthetics, we should be guilty of deception and dishonesty towards the woman when she has made a great effort to control the process of labour so that she can bring the child into the world through her own action.

C.W.P. demands certain conditions—economic and social. Money is needed, and the method must be strictly adhered to. If not it will soon be said that C.W.P. is not giving results, and women—either ignorant or not vigilant enough—will suffer because the method will be abandoned.

C.W.P., as Dr. Lamaze often said, is women's greatest victory. Our generation must strengthen it for those who come after us. Pope Pius XII made his attitude clear and explained the position of the Church vis-à-vis psychoprophylaxis. He understood the method and did not confuse it with others.

We are often asked if every woman who has been well prepared can give birth without pain. We say no. It is a French idea to offer C.W.P. training to all women who want it. Dr. Lamaze took a great risk when he decided to do this. He was quite right—for the women are then unselected. We teach every woman that childbirth is a normal physiological phenomenon. Even women who cannot expect complete success—those with abnormal pelvises, for example—can benefit from the training. It acts as a premedication before operation and brings an additional sense of security during pregnancy.

If we had wanted to produce even more convincing statistics, we could have trained only suitable cases. But then we could not have created a public opinion which is the method's strongest support.

We divide women into three groups:

1. *Normal cases.* There is a normal pelvis, good presentation of the baby (head well flexed, or even a breech), good physical and psychological conditions. The woman can expect childbirth without any pain, provided that no family, money or social worries upset her just before the birth. This group contains about forty per cent of women.

2. *On the borderline of normality.* The pregnancy has developed normally. Obstetrical examinations have indicated that confinement will be normal. The training is good. But there may be mechanical difficulties—the head too engaged, producing false labour during the two or three days before confinement; the confinement itself occurring too quickly; the head not completely flexed; the cervix not soft enough; the uterus containing a small fibroma which causes some irregularity

of contraction. The difficulties will affect the activity of the uterus, both in contraction and relaxation.

In many cases excellent childbirth may be achieved. The better the mental equilibrium of the woman, the better will be the result. But we must try to keep labour as normal as possible by the use of medicine in very small—almost homeopathic—doses.

If we did not do this we should end in certain failure. The woman in this group needs to be helped, but at the same time her training will stand her in good stead. From 40 to 45 per cent of women are in this group. Although there are small difficulties, all, or nearly all, will be able to satisfy their deep desire to bring their babies into the world by themselves—fully conscious. With these women the doctor or the midwife must have a complete knowledge of the method.

The first two groups represent, therefore, 80 to 85 per cent of women. They benefit from C.W.P. without any use of anaesthetics— except the use of language.

3. *Abnormal Cases.* Here the doctor must be experienced and the woman perfectly trained and understanding. The psychoprophylactic method will allow her to bear a difficult confinement that otherwise she could not stand. The doctor can carry out longer trial labour (four to six hours in some cases); can avoid forceps or make a forceps delivery easy when otherwise it would have been difficult, and can use forceps in cases where a Caesarian section might have been necessary. In a remarkable way the method may reduce symptoms pointing to a Caesarian operation. Possibly 12 to 15 per cent of women are in this group.

Even if an operation is necessary, the woman will face it calmly because she understands the reasons for it. So the anaesthetic will be reduced to a minimum, which will be a great advantage to her and her baby.

The dramatic cases in obstetrics, such as placenta praevia or prolapse of the cord, lie outside psychoprophylaxis because they are pathological.

It is obvious that complete confidence must exist between the woman and the doctor or midwife. But this confidence must not be only an emotional relationship; it must be founded on knowledge.

4

Read's Theory

In France the method of Dr. G. Dick Read is often confused with psychoprophylaxis. On the other hand the two are sometimes contrasted.

Read's work must be placed in its historical context—the period between the two wars (1919 to 1940). He worked alone to defend his ideas, which are now recognized as valuable in obstetrics and to the world in general. We ourselves pay tribute to him. His work has a definite place in a study of verbal analgesia in obstetrics, but it seems to us only an important step towards psychoprophylaxis—as indeed have been the works of the French and Russian schools on suggestion and hypnosis.

Dr. Dick Read thinks that pain in childbirth is by no means inevitable, but that any negative emotion such as fear of childbirth engenders it. His clinical and psychological knowledge, combined with daily observation of women in labour, has led him to believe that many psychological factors increase the pain in childbirth. These include: mental tiredness, heightened by loneliness and ignorance of labour; inadequate behaviour of doctor or midwife; unsuitable atmosphere in the maternity home and other factors. 'The mask, the gown, the rubber gloves, expectant searching down below and quiet steps awaken in a woman's mind a host of fears and doubts.' (*Childbirth without Fear*)

Read regards fear as one of the main causes of pain. Fear is a burdensome heritage handed down from generation to generation and kept up by books, newspapers, radio and cinema—which flourishes in the absence of sexual and obstetrical education. He blames civilization for its evil influence on women's minds.

He refers to Pavlov in his interpretation of the physiological mechanisms of fear in relation to childbirth, but he does not explore the field of conditioned reflexes. Fear causes, he thinks, disharmony in the working of the uterus, and this becomes painful.

How can fear be overcome? By antenatal training which will diminish the disastrous effects of civilization, and bring the act of birth back to its primitive state. Dr. Read uses muscular relaxation to combat the tension created by fear. 'Therefore fear, pain and tension are the three evils which are not normal to the natural design, but which have been introduced in the course of civilization by the ignorance of those who have been concerned with attendance at childbirth.'

If pain, fear and tension go hand in hand, tension must be relieved and fear overcome to eliminate pain.

Studying Read's work, one regrets that he stopped here, and did not try to penetrate more deeply into the nature of fear and pain. He has not formulated a comprehensive theory on the origin of pain in childbirth and so has not found a coherent method of combating it.

The antenatal training that he gives is rather vague—not as precise as in psychoprophylaxis. Mysticism frequently borders on mechanism. He considers gymnastics very important for curing 'the weakness of the abdominal muscles'!

Dr. Read separates psychological from somatic activity. He considers that the more the work of the uterus is outside a woman's consciousness, the more natural it will be and therefore painless. 'The partial consciousness, the temporary loss of control by the brain, thus allow the expulsive activities to work unimpaired.'

To summarize we suggest that Dr. Read has dealt too empirically with the problem of pain. He has not sufficiently studied the deep mechanisms as psychoprophylaxis tries to do. He does not sufficiently take into account the close and constant bond between mind and body. Between his ideas and those of Pavlov's school there is a fundamental difference. He gives the woman a passive rôle through dilatation, while psychoprophylaxis gives her as much activity as possible throughout labour.

Dr. Read's work seems to us very interesting. It is the work of an isolated individual fighting critics who possess neither his generosity nor his human qualities. Here is one account:

Mrs. T.

I gave birth on 28 June to my third child, a boy weighing 8 lb. 6½ oz., and I did not suffer at all after I had reached the clinic and could start the method of childbirth without pain.

I had not thought previously that it could be completely successful —except in somewhat rare privileged cases. I thought it would not work for me. I had no confidence either in the method or myself. I knew only one person in France who had tried it. She had had a conscientious training and did her best, but she could not suppress the pain completely—only lessen it. And I had had my first two babies in Sydney, where all the nursing-homes have for several years used a method of 'childbirth without fear', which they claim to be Dr. Read's. In practice it is very different from the French method.

During the training, which consists of gymnastics and relaxation exercises, and also some explanation of pregnancy and childbirth, you are not taught how to breathe or push. You are warned that you will have pain during confinement, but that it will be bearable and that you will be able to bring your baby into the world without an anaesthetic.

During confinement a rather primitive method is used. It consists of deep breathing exercises during contractions and relaxation exercises. During delivery you are just asked to push, but without stopping breathing and with any kind of action, so that, although the pain is less, it is still far from eliminated.

The psychological aspect is completely neglected. The husband is not allowed to be present at the childbirth. The assistant or nurse who has done the training is not there. When the dilatation period is lengthy you are left alone for long periods. The nurses do not take any notice of contractions, nor give you medical care at any time. The labour wards are not private, or, if they are, the doors are left open so that you can see and hear what is happening in the others. And the nurses make no effort to hide their indifference.

Yet the method seemed interesting, for it allows the woman to take part in the birth of her baby, to accept the pains of childbirth and have the great joy of being conscious when the baby is born. But my experience had convinced me that it was practically impossible to remove childbirth pains completely.

All this explains why I was not very confident before this third birth. I was also rather tired at the end of my pregnancy, and I was afraid of not having enough energy to make the effort needed in childbirth without pain. This fatigue had prevented me from doing the breathing and pushing exercises regularly. My training was, in fact, only four sessions with my assistant and two or three by myself at home.

And, finally, I could not help thinking about my second childbirth, which had been rather difficult. Delivery had lasted an hour, and the pains remained very strong, though I pushed as much as I could at each contraction.

During the last weeks of pregnancy I felt apprehensive though I tried not to. But in spite of worry I was determined to use the method as conscientiously as possible. I was anxious not to be anaesthetized when the baby was born.

Labour started on 28 June at 5 a.m.—not with contractions but a dull continuous pain in the back. At about 8.30 a.m. I felt the first contraction, very strong and prolonged, which was followed by another after an hour. In the interim I again felt a dull pain in back and also stomach. It was easily bearable as long as I was lying down, but very painful as soon as I tried to get up. At 9.30 a.m. came another contraction similar to the first. As I had lost no blood, water nor the mucous plug, I preferred to wait a bit longer before telephoning to the clinic. At last, about ten o'clock, regular contractions began, very close together—about every 2½ minutes. I then telephoned Mlle H. and the clinic. I must have arrived at about 10.30 a.m. I was already at the end of dilatation, and was able to begin the method. Contractions were very close and strong, but did not last very long.

I found this the most difficult period of childbirth. I managed to get rid of pain by quick breathing and by emptying my mind of thought and memory—concentrating only on breathing. But I felt the contractions vividly as a sensation which was not painful but was rather like the pain of contractions in my previous childbirths. I felt I was only just succeeding in avoiding pain; the least thing could have upset my psychological equilibrium. What helped me most was the habit I had acquired during my pregnancy of not thinking, of emptying my mind as I trained myself to muscular relaxation. At the required moment I was able to concentrate on something definite, which happened to be the quick respiration. But I should not have succeeded very well alone. The presence of my assistant was most valuable. She provided what was lacking in me. Also, this difficult period was short, and so the effort was easier to make.

At about eleven the doctor arrived. He immediately ruptured the membranes. It did not hurt at all, and I was relieved to think that I was starting the last stage of labour. I was placed in position for delivery, and was told that at the next contraction I could push. As soon as I felt the contraction coming I told the doctor who then directed me completely—'Breathe. Stop breathing. Push. Breathe out. Breathe in. Stop breathing' and so on. To my great surprise I found that in this way I could avoid not only all pain but the very sensation of the contraction. That was a great relief, as I had for a long time been afraid of this period of delivery, which I thought the most painful. After the effort of dilatation, the pushing seemed far easier and very nice.

As the baby's head was not in a good position, the doctor decided to put it into place with forceps. I felt nothing when he used the first, but the second pinched me unexpectedly and I screamed. During the next contraction, while I was pushing, the doctor changed the position of the head and I felt nothing.

After I had pushed a bit more, the head stopped at the vulva, stretching the perineum and producing an easily bearable tugging feeling. The doctor, after letting me recover breath, made me push without waiting for a contraction, and at last the head came out. I pushed again to deliver the shoulders. This was quite painless. It felt only like something soft coming through. And at last I could see the baby, who was put on my stomach. I was enormously relieved that everything had gone so quickly and well, and I felt the great joy that I suppose every mother feels at seeing her baby for the first time.

After ten minutes the placenta was delivered without trouble. Then the doctor, assistant and midwife left me alone with my husband. But I felt so tired that for a good half hour I lost my happiness and was only aware of exhaustion. But luckily this feeling did not last long. At about noon lunch was brought, and I quickly recovered strength and good spirits.

I can make no criticism of the method, which seemed perfect. Of course it does demand some effort, but every possible help was given me to produce it. Everything seemed minutely controlled, and this attention to the smallest detail seemed one of the important factors. Everything went like a well-run-in machine, and this increased my confidence in the others and myself. And I was thankful for the calm and quiet of the labour ward, the attention that assistant and midwife gave to contractions, everyone's kindness and good humour and the presence of my husband. I felt that I was being helped all the time, not only physically but morally.

The assistant's part seems very important. During training a human contact is made, so that at childbirth, instead of feeling strange on arrival at the clinic, you feel that you are being helped by someone who knows you and is interested in you.

The doctor's attitude is also important. An indifferent, worried, bored or too serious attitude could spoil everything. I liked the doctor's good humour and briskness. This created a relaxed happy atmosphere which helped me a lot.

The method brought me more than the mere suppression of pain. It made the confinement one of the best moments of my life. Most important for the mother is her voluntary joyful co-operation in the birth of the child. In a traditional birth it is rather terrible to feel that a whole mechanism has been set going which you have not wanted and cannot control. The woman's instinctive reaction is to resist the process which is taking place without her consent and is going to hurt her. Her baby's birth seems secondary, and her most immediate desire is to stop the process. Instead of relaxing, so that labour can go on, she becomes tense.

In childbirth without pain, on the other hand, she accepts the mechanism. She works with the labour, instead of resisting it. She controls it and really feels that she is taking part in the baby's birth— which she wants. Instead of being hostile to what is happening inside her, or just passive, she feels that she is bringing her baby into the world instead of waiting for it to come by itself. This active participation is extremely stimulating.

Then, when all goes well, you are conscious of achieving—with the doctor, midwife, assistant and your husband—good teamwork, and that gives satisfaction. Finally—and this has a greater effect than all the rest—there is the presence of your husband. He has taken an interest in the training, discussed it with you during pregnancy, and then he gives you the help of his presence at the actual birth. This makes the bonds even stronger between a couple. They have had extra experience together; their marriage has brought great richness.

PART TWO

THE COMPLETE TRAINING FOR CHILDBIRTH WITHOUT PAIN

Lecture 1

Preliminary Lecture to the Husbands

IRST of all, I am going to speak to the husbands, the fathers. A few years ago I went through a similar time—waiting for the birth of a baby. For nine months I heard all the things that you are likely to hear—advice, technical details, discussion on whether it will be a boy or a girl, jokes about being a father, the duties and obligations which go with childbirth, what one must and must not do, what the neighbours think, what uncle, grandmother and everybody else think.

This wait during his wife's pregnancy is not really difficult for the husband, but it is somewhat ridiculous, and in any case it is a nuisance. Now we are going to see if we cannot completely change this situation.

Do not think that, through some amazing discovery, the man will be able to help his wife by bearing the child himself, like the male sea-horse. If that were so, it would no longer be possible to make the bitter remark which you have certainly heard: 'Ah, men! It's not you who have to bear children!'

It is true, we do not bear children. But what is the good of complaining about that? We are facing fact. Being useful to a woman means helping her, not looking on or pitying her. So we must examine critically the old, generally accepted ideas concerning the social phenomenon of maternity.

Why did it often happen that, although they did not always express it in words, a man and woman became antagonistic after he had shown his love for her? It was as if the sexes became charged with electricity after intercourse and repelled each other. How did it happen that the union, desired and freely realized in the act of love, did not afterwards follow its natural course?

This breach occurred because the conscious participation by the couple in the act of transmitting life ceased with the completion of the

39

act. Then they began a long entirely passive period of waiting. The woman was 'carrying,' as it was so crudely put. Her abdomen became more obvious, while she (perhaps knitting in front of it) tried to conceal it. The husband looked at his wife, admiring her as a courageous person who undertakes a difficult task without flinching, and there was nothing else they could do.

Ignorance once more exerted its paralysing influence. It produced a passive attitude.

The woman was entitled, as is any animal, to the natural protection of the male. But she was not entitled to as much attention, care, supervision and active help as a plant. Let us consider the farmer. After sowing his seed, he takes pride in the corn as it grows. He looks after his grain, adds fertilizer, weeds his soil and clears it of parasites. He knows that the more care he takes of it, the richer, the stronger and the more beautiful his produce will be. His land, fields, trees, plants, vines and corn—he loves them all. He can improve them because he knows them so well. He knows what they need just as he knows what they can do. He has watched them and studied them. He bends over to attend to them, and the earth and its fruits give him his reward.

This comparison is no doubt superficial. But it is applicable to man. And we are going to see how a husband and wife can co-operate consciously in the task of maternity.

Because of their almost complete ignorance of what happens in pregnancy and childbirth, the man and woman cannot help themselves. The woman feels vaguely that something should be done; that the circumstances of her pregnancy might have been improved—and not only its medical aspects. She is going to add a human life to society but, on account of her pregnancy, is isolated and regarded as a person apart. And the world shows kind but ineffectual concern. Her husband the family, friends and strangers—everyone is considerate and talks a lot, but nobody does anything.

No indeed! It is not only a matter of concern, respect, kind words and good will.

Because it is a social phenomenon, maternity involves all members of society. If the phenomenon is understood everybody can make a contribution, and the father's part especially will no longer be limited to a momentary organic function.

After all, when women used to say ironically that we got nothing but pleasure from this experience, they were not completely wrong.

The man was somewhat like those warriors who, in the old days, came back from the war and gave their wives babies. Those medieval customs have brought their worries, which are sometimes serious. Wives think about us from time to time but with a severity as strong as the tenderness with which they previously welcomed us.

The days pass.

As confinement draws near, what dignity we have left has vanished in the rising excitement which takes hold of the family. The doctors and nurses are bombarded with questions, which are often absurd. Their answers are no better. The husband is considered a nuisance, harmful, laden with germs. It is said ironically that he goes through more than his wife.

At last, in an atmosphere of grave anxiety, though in spite of everything there is a feeling of joy, the happy event takes place. We are all delivered, freed of a worry nine months old.

The mother is alive; baby alive; father too. The doctor comes through it well.

The father forgets the difficult days when he waited helplessly. Overcome with emotion, he determines to be an angel to everybody. He is congratulated by his family and friends. One of them says inevitably, 'Your baby? He's the living image of me'—and everyone laughs.

Although happiness should not be excluded from our present ideas, the man and the woman who create a new being assume rights and duties. The woman has not only rights. The man has not only duties. We believe that mutual participation in the events of maternity will provide a solid basis for the couple's relationship. It will improve the conditions in which life is passed on, and, even more, the well-being of the baby. Society and the individual will gain from each other. This mutual gain is founded on knowledge.

There is no need to philosophize. Organized action is open to us; it will improve our lives. Let us take advantage of it.

The husband is the closest person to his wife in her immediate circle. It is he who exerts the strongest, most frequent and lasting influence upon her. In general, the more he knows, the more valuable his influence will be.

This is what we suggest that you should do during your wife's pregnancy:

1. Attend the course of lectures given to the wives.

The training starts now at the beginning of pregnancy. The

lectures are far apart, and you can arrange to be free for them. We ask you to suggest suitable days and times.

2. If this is impossible, become familiar with the psychoprophylactic method with the help of your wife. This will be an excellent way for her to revise it.

3. In any case, add to what you know by reading what is published about it.

4. Get an idea of the practical aspects, checking the results obtained by your wife when carrying out the exercises.

You can do this best and understand the exercises properly only if you practise them yourselves. We advise you to compare results and to discuss and criticize them. You should try all the time to think of the exercises in relation to pregnancy and childbirth in order to understand their use and significance thoroughly. They must never be done automatically. All the exercises should be thought out.

Then, during childbirth, the father will be the most helpful person present. He will notice mistakes which can then be corrected.

5. We strongly recommend that you, with your wife, should look carefully for all signs indicating life in your baby—in particular, the baby's movements, how strong they are in different stages of the pregnancy, their extent, how often they occur and how long they last.

Also, you should listen to the heart beats. In this way you will be the second witness of your baby's life and of his first movements. You will feel his presence although he is still invisible.

6. You will help your wife finally by observing with her the contractions of the uterus, the hollow muscle with contains the baby. When they become regular, these contractions will mark the beginning of childbirth. You appreciate that the more she understands them, the more easily will she react and adapt to them.

Then her behaviour will depend partly upon you. You will experience her confinement with her. With her, too, you will hear your baby's first cry.

The first two lectures deal with fertilization and the development of the egg until term. We explain how the mother can get used to her new situation.

Towards the fifth month of pregnancy we give an account of the principles of the psychoprophylactic method. It is a theoretical lecture.

Then follows a lecture on respiration and its anatomical and physiological relationship with some of the reproductive organs.

One lecture is on neuro-muscular training. Two lectures deal with what the woman should do during dilatation and delivery. Finally, there is a recapitulation accompanied by practical revision and a visit to the maternity centre.

The teaching which is given to you for your benefit is not entirely elementary. So we advise you to take notes during the lectures. This is the best way to memorize them. These notes will always be useful to you. When you come back to see us, expecting another baby, you will be able to make comparisons. The principles will still be the same, but, as experience increases, we shall make progress with our techniques.

As Dr. Lamaze said: 'The method is constantly evolving.'

Lecture 2

Fertilization and the First Three Months
of Development

THOUGH we have forgotten much that we learnt at school, we can still remember the story of the successive changes in the frog or butterfly before it reaches its final form. We know its metamorphoses—from the egg of the butterfly, for example, which first becomes a larva, then a pupa and finally the perfect insect. We were all deeply interested in these transformations from something which seemed inanimate to a living thing. It is, no doubt, the movement, the life in these metamorphoses which arouses our interest and holds our attention.

Life is indeed characterized by movement. The interest, mixed with emotion, with which we follow the first steps of the baby is related to the actual movement by which a living being adapts himself to his conditions of life.

Sometimes, we are tempted to say that animals, insects and amphibia are superior to us because they can live without help as soon as they arrive in the world. Since we are born not quite in our final form, we must, in order to survive, turn towards those who came before us for sustenance and protection. For us there is no metamorphosis, no larval state. Although we cannot survive alone, at least we have the pride of possessing at birth almost the form which we shall keep; the pride, too, of knowing that our powers of adaptation will be greater than that of animals. And we ourselves do undergo metamorphosis. Also, although we cannot look after ourselves from the start, the organism which creates us can himself look after us, whereas in the lower orders this is not so.

And these differences are the result of a slow evolution of species over millions of years, evolution related to different needs as times changed.

44

As Dr. Haeckel said: 'Few people realize that man, in the course of his development, goes through a series of transformations just as amazing as the familiar metamorphoses of the butterfly.' This ignorance has arisen because the metamorphoses take place in the mother's womb. We cannot see them.

Nevertheless the means of investigation which science has put into our hands have gradually enabled us to recognize them, study them and learn from them, though we are far from understanding what are called 'the mysteries of life'.

And today, we are going to tell you what we know of the metamorphoses which have been going on inside your body for the last few weeks.

One day, a single cell among millions of others in the extraordinary 'living liquid,' of which Jean Rostand spoke, flowed into you. After travelling quickly over a long and difficult course, this cell, which is called a spermatozoon, at last reached its destination. Then it met a cell much bigger than itself, penetrated it and fused with it. From this fertilization of the ovule, a human being like you and me will later develop.

But let us look closely at the beginning and end of the process. These two tiny cells, completely invisible to the naked eye, will fuse and form one. Then they will proliferate and multiply; and when the human being is formed, finished, do you know how many cells he will be made of? One hundred thousand billion.

Whether there is one cell or one hundred thousand billion cells, each is organized. It lives, moves, feeds, excretes, burns energy, takes up oxygen and responds to stimuli. But it is obvious that the mode of organization differs greatly from one part to another.

After the head of the spermatozoon has fused with the nucleus of the ovule, the fertilized ovum or egg is formed. Straight away it begins to respire intensely. Its oxygen consumption (O_2) is greatly increased as its temperature rises. The male and female cells met in one of the two Fallopian tubes found one on each side of the upper part of the uterus. Through these tubes, the ovules produced by the ovaries reach the uterine cavity.

When the ovule is not fertilized, it dies and is absorbed. At the same time, the mucous membrane of the uterus—which had become congested and swollen as if ready to receive an egg—disintegrates and bleeds. That is why Jean Rostand says: 'Woman pays with her blood each month for failing to conceive.'

But let us return to the fertilized ovule. The egg passes through the Fallopian tube into the uterine cavity. During this migration, it is not inactive. It begins to divide and wastes no time. The divisions start very simply. The first cell divides into two cells. Each of these itself produces two other cells and so on.

At that time, the egg is a sphere with an irregular surface. It resembles a mulberry. This is why it was called *morula*.[1] The cell multiplication continues. The cells do not increase in volume, but they become arranged in a very definite way. On the surface of the sphere, small cells form a layer; they ensure the nourishment of all the cells. Inside, the cells are bigger and are massed together. The egg, truly alive, moves towards the uterus. At this stage, it lives on itself, drawing on its own reserves.

When the egg consists of sixty-four cells, it can no longer support itself. And to ensure the life of the cells, which continue to multiply unflaggingly and are now getting larger, it resorts to the substance in which it is bathed. It thus converts the food it absorbs into human components.

After travelling for about eight days, it reaches the uterine cavity where it is going to stay and have full board and lodging for a long time. We say that it becomes embedded, and this occurs right in the uterine mucosa which is swollen, soft, hypertrophied and congested. It benefits immediately from the richness of the lining of the uterus. Our traveller has a hearty appetite when he reaches the end of the journey, and he satisfies his needs ravenously, gaining sustenance from nearby vessels. The egg is only the size of the head of a pin; nevertheless, an oval spot becomes visible on its surface. It is the embryonic disc, which, in the egg, is the origin of the future man.

To imagine better what the embryo is like, we can look at a hen's egg, where, in the yolk, we have all noticed a reddish streak—the germ.

To summarize:

1. A female cell is fertilized by a male cell. These two cells fuse and form only one cell. This is the egg.

2. The egg develops. The cells multiply. They are arranged in a sphere in two layers:

an internal layer (endoblast) and
an external layer (trophoblast).

3. The primitive streak appears on the internal layer. From then on, the metamorphoses begin. The embryo, as we have just seen, is

---

[1] μορον = mulberry.

not formed from the whole egg but from a part only. Inside, the primitive streak is thus itself formed of two layers of superimposed cells.

Soon a third layer of cells develops between them. Each of these three layers will give rise to well-defined tissues in our body. From the first layer, which is called the *endoderm*, will develop the digestive tract, the respiratory apparatus, the liver, the thyroid and the pancreas. From the second layer, called the *ectoderm*, will develop the nervous system, the special sense organs and the skin. From the intermediate layer, or *mesoderm*, will develop the circulatory system, the skeleton, the muscles and the kidneys.

So that we have in the order of their appearance, which is related to the embryo's needs:

1. The tissues immediately necessary for life: the digestive tract.

2. The tissues for the protection and organization of a structure rapidly becoming complex; the nervous system, the skin.

3. The tissues which will maintain the shape and the architecture of the whole.

Before discussing in detail the sequence of changes in the embryo, we should describe how its life is made secure—how it obtains nourishment and takes up oxygen.

The human egg, unlike the hen's egg, is almost completely without reserves of food. The mother must therefore support it. The exchanges between the mother and the egg occur indirectly.

As a rule, the egg becomes embedded in the wall of the upper part of the uterus. Its implantation in the uterine mucosa results from the digestive properties of the peripheral cells. A process of branching occurs, and gradually a mass forms between the mother and the egg. It is the *placenta*, which extends into a cord containing two arteries and a vein—the *umbilical cord*.

Physiologically, the placenta is very important. It prevents the maternal blood from passing directly to the foetus. It collects the maternal blood and, at the same time, reduces its pressure and speed. It is not an ordinary filter, and substances are probably made in it and chemical reactions brought about in it. The composition of maternal blood is in fact different from foetal blood. It allows antibodies to pass through; on the other hand, it prevents many germs from crossing. It secretes hormones. Through it the necessities of life are provided for the egg.

We can now resume the story of metamorphoses. About fifteen

days after fertilization, a dark line appears in the middle of the embry-onic disc. It is the neural groove, the beginning of the nervous system. The groove deepens, and soon its upper edges join. At the end of the fifth week, the tube, where the spinal cord will form, is closed; its anterior end hypertrophies. The brain is taking shape. The dorsal part of the embryo will become the back. The growth of the cells is parti-cularly important in this region, for it gives the embryo its rounded, spherical shape. It doubles over itself. On each side of the tube, minute bulges can soon be seen, and when the tube is completely closed, forty-one pairs of these can be counted. They will be the vertebrae.

When it is one month old, the strange animal that is the embryo is about a quarter of an inch long. It is made up of roughly three parts or rather three swellings. The most important is the cephalic enlargement, which at that time occupies more than a third of the total volume. What will be the head is already outlined. Laterally the eyes take on a rough shape. The ear is indicated by a mark; the nose by a hole and the jaw by a prominence.

In the middle of the embryonic mass the chest will develop. We can make out the important swellings formed by the heart and liver. The heart and circulation, at this stage of development, look like the heart and circulation of the fish, from which it is said we are derived. The circulation, although rudimentary, exists. The heart lives and pumps the blood which reaches it at an extremely low pressure. The organism is living.

Until it is four weeks old, the future human being has neither legs nor arms. These will appear during the fifth week in the form of buds.

Development continues, except posteriorly. The end portion, prolonging so to speak the spine to form a tail, will disappear.

During the seventh week, the neck is formed and the animal straightens out a little. The facial features become more definite. It is a strange face with a surprised expression. The eyes are wide open, without eyelids. The forehead and the skull are enormous. The brain already contains millions and millions of cells.

The embryo has reflexes; swallowing and suction. It moves, but its movements are weak and unordered. Its circulatory system has become more complicated. It is almost what it will be at birth. The cartilages, which help to maintain the shape, are hardening. The centres of ossification appear. Towards the fiftieth day the clavicle starts things off. In fifteen more days, the one hundred and ten pieces, or there-abouts, of our skeleton will be ossified.

Towards and during the course of the third month, the foetus produces its own red and white cells with the help of the liver. It is beginning to depend less on its mother. This is proved by the perfecting of its circulatory system and especially its heart. The excretory organs, in particular the kidneys, take up their positions and assume their final shape. It is interesting to observe that our eventual kidneys are derived from two other kidneys of totally different structure and shape.

From the eighth week, we speak of the foetus, because from then on the embryo possess the shape of the human species. If it were expelled from the uterus, it could live for a few hours. And one could easily identify it as a girl or a boy.

You know now how fertilization occurs, how the embryo forms and how it develops until it becomes a foetus. We have said nothing about the mother, nothing about the body which makes the birth of the baby possible.

The woman's body undergoes many changes. We could almost say that new functions are created. We will go into all this in detail in the next lecture.

Today, we will only point out that these changes are both chemical and physical and that the proper working of our organs depends on the nervous system.

Chemical changes occur since the maintenance of the baby, during its growth in the uterus, involves very important new requirements, particularly oxygen, without which combustion, reaction and organic oxidation cannot occur.

Physical changes also take place. They are not very pleasant for the woman. We begin very early to teach you certain exercises. We want to prevent the inconveniences which used to accompany bodily changes during pregnancy.

The training you will receive helps to maintain nervous equilibrium. The breathing exercises will improve the ventilation of your lungs and will provide plenty of oxygen for the needs of your organs. They will prevent excessive curvature of the vertebral column. They will increase or maintain the tone of your abdominal muscles. They will help very effectively to keep up a healthy venous circulation, particularly in the legs.

Thus, the fear, which is sometimes profound in pregnant women, of losing their mental equilibrium, and of seeing their health and strength affected, the fear that they cannot do their work, and meet their social obligations, will disappear. So will the idea of the expectant mother as an extremely delicate person, who must wear low-heeled shoes, and a special belt, eat enough for two, not cross her legs and read light books. These antiquated ideas, fears, and worries, which resulted from inactivity produced and permitted by ignorance, will give way to a rational training in which we combine theory and practice. It is of this that prophylaxis—prevention—consists.

EXERCISES

1. *In a semi-recumbent position* (for example in a deck chair), arms alongside the body, breathing. Without straining, *breathe in*, palms upwards, *breathe out*, palms turned downwards, slightly lifting the head. Imagine that you blow a candle to disturb the flame without putting it out. At the same time, contract the muscles of the buttocks. If possible, do this morning and night for five minutes.

2. *In a semi-recumbent position*, legs extended but relaxed, externally rotate the legs and feet, slowly. Internally rotate the legs, and feet, slowly. Ten times each leg.

3. Every morning, between getting up and breakfast or dressing, walk on the tips of your toes. Do not exceed ten minutes.

Lecture 3

From the Fourth Month until Term

WHEN the foetus enters its fourth month, it has the rudiments of all the organs that will make a human being. From then on they will be completed and perfected.

The period from the fourth month until term is characterized by:

1. The importance assumed by the nervous system, particularly the brain.

2. Foetal movements, showing that the baby is alive.

3. The increase in weight, size and volume of the foetus.

Let us now study these points in detail.

The Importance of the Nervous System

Touch, movement, sensory perception, all our connexions with the environment in which we live, depend on our nervous system which can at the same time receive, intercept, transmit, analyse, synthesize, and respond—functions which it can also fulfil for the internal organs, thus regulating their activity. Only a nervous system which has reached the highest degree of perfection can undertake such a rôle.

We have seen that it takes shape very early in the embryo. The extremely rapid development of the dorsal part of the embryo makes it curve. It has been said of the characteristic position of the foetus that it tries to take up as little room as possible. This posture is maintained by the baby for several months after birth.

But, of the whole nervous system, it is obviously the brain which grows the most rapidly. The strange appearance of the foetus is due to this disproportion between the head and the rest of the body. At birth the head weighs 12 oz. in a baby of 6 lb. which is an eighth of the total weight.

By virtue of his brain, man is the animal which adapts best to his environment. We shall expand this subject in the next lecture.

Morphologically, it is the frontal region which, because of its size, especially differentiates the brain of man from that of the animal. Although big and weighing so much, and although all its cells are present, the brain of the new-born is not yet ready to assume all its responsibilities. It is not finished, neither is the nervous system as a whole. The cells which make it up have not yet reached maturity. The cerebral cortex is not yet excitable; it is believed that sensation is not consciously appreciated at birth.

The nervous system of a child is very delicate and rapidly becomes exhausted. The baby needs many hours of sleep during the first months of life. Certain parts of his brain are not fully developed, in particular those which co-ordinate movements and give them precision. We have all observed how clumsy a child is. We have also noticed that he complains very quickly if he has to stand still or walk for any length of time. We say that he is pretending, and point out that, once back home, he will fidget, jump and dance about and not be tired any more.

All this is true. But the child is not pretending. Walking tires him, but jumping, dancing, crouching, rushing and rolling do not.

We cannot ask for either a prolonged or repetitive effort from particular parts of a child's nervous system because exhaustion occurs very quickly. If the movements are not varied, there is exhaustion, but it does not occur if the movements are varied.

One more word about the nervous system. We often hear it said of a child: 'He learned to walk very young.' Certainly not! We do not learn to walk. We walk when it has become physiologically possible.

At birth, as we have just said, the baby is curled up. He keeps this position for a long time. He first uses his four limbs for movement's sake. We say that the neuromuscular tone is uppermost in the flexors, which means that the child can easily flex his thighs on his pelvis and his calves on his thighs. The opposite is impossible for him. He cannot stand upright because he cannot extend his legs. The development of his nervous system will allow the extensors to take precedence; his legs will be able to extend, and walking will become possible.

Movements of the foetus

This is the second important feature of pregnancy between the fourth month and term. The foetus moves well before the fourth month, but these movements cannot be felt. At the fourth month, the arms and legs are well developed. The muscular system takes shape. The foetus becomes stronger; his movements are then active enough to be felt.

Towards four and a half months the beating of the heart can be heard. The circulation has become vigorous, and the cardiac rhythm is about 130 to 150 beats per minute. It is said that the heart of a boy beats more strongly and slowly.

The circulation of the blood is not the same as in the new-born. The oxygenation of the blood does not depend on the lungs, which are not included in the circulation. It is not until birth that important changes take place, in particular in the heart and in certain vessels, enabling the child to gain complete control of its own supply of oxygen.

The increase in weight, size and volume of the foetus

As the circulation of the foetus becomes stronger, his weight and size increase. We will give you some surprising figures.

When it is formed, the egg is invisible to the naked eye. It measures must less then one fiftieth of an inch.

At the end of the first month, the embryo is about a quarter of an inch long.

At the end of the second month, the embryo is about one inch long.

At the end of the third month, its length is about four inches.

At term the baby is about twenty inches long.

Its development is therefore more rapid at the beginning. The cell divisions are, in fact, easier and more frequent at the beginning. Later they entail more and more elaborate organization. They are then slower and more laborious. Some biologists say also that this is a sign of growing old—already.

The increase in weight is still more amazing. The egg would weigh less than one sixtieth of a grain; the baby at birth 7 lb. The foetus is contained in an organ formed mainly of muscular tissue, which as we know already is called the uterus. This, when not in use, weighs about 2 oz. In a woman at term it weighs about $2\frac{1}{2}$ lb. The placenta weighs just over 1 lb.; the amniotic fluid between $\frac{1}{2}$ lb. and 2 lb. That is a total average increase of about 12 lb.

Now we know that the increase in weight of a pregnant woman, as a rule, greatly exceeds this figure; it lies between 9 lb. and 26 lb. The difference is added by the woman herself. The mother's body undergoes varied and important changes.

The following changes are chemical:

The production of hormones. Some increase; others decrease or disappear.

The laying down of fat. We lay it down better than we get rid of it, so there is no need to eat for two.

The transmission of calcium. The baby's skeleton forms at the mother's expense. But do not imagine that this calcium leaves the mother's bones to be transplanted into the bone of the developing foetus—in the same way as we collect sand for the walls of a house. The calcium produced by the mother is diverted. They are two consumers: the smaller of the two is by far the harder to please.

The composition of the urine. This contains certain products through which pregnancy can be detected very early on.

Finally, to defend herself against the toxic products secreted by the egg when it is embedded as early as the first week, the mother must produce what are called antibodies—products capable of neutralizing these toxins.

The activity of the nervous system increases, keeping even the least important of our organs and their functions under control.

These new needs and extra work of the woman's body are associated with an increased demand of O_2. And here we have the first reason for the breathing exercises that we ask you to do. They will improve the ventilation of your lungs.

But there are also physical and mechanical changes.

The baby occupies the uterus, which is in the abdominal cavity; together, the uterus and the fluid weigh, we have said, about 12 lb. This weight is a force which acts at the level of the pelvis very much in front of the axis on which the pelvis rests. The pelvis is balanced in upright position on the bones of the thighs—the femurs. The pelvis can, as a result, turn or tilt to a certain extent on the axis of rotation formed by the hip joint.

In the pregnant woman, the pelvis tilts from the back to the front and from above downwards. The pubis is drawn downwards slightly and the hips forwards. The vertebral column, fixed to the pelvis, obviously follows this movement. The normal curves increase. The lumbar region is hollowed out from the back to the front. Your back arches, the dorsal region bows from front to back to restore the balance, and you have a rounder back.

The increase in the lumbar curve is usually accompanied by rapid fatigue and pains which may extend along the sciatic nerve. The compensatory increase in the dorsal curve also means tiredness and pains, but above all difficulty in breathing. Nearly all pregnant women complain of this trouble, which is naturally even more obvious in women suffering from diseases of the respiratory system.

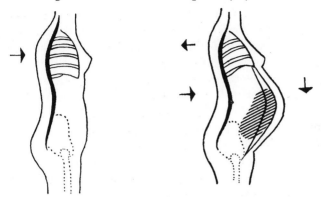

This difficulty is easily explained. When the curve of the dorsal vertebrae increases, the contact of the joints between the vertebrae slightly alters, and, hence, that of the joints between the vertebrae and the ribs is also modified, so that the ribs no longer move freely. The range of the thoracic movements is reduced. The expansion of the lungs dependent on it is also reduced. The result—fatigue, pains and less oxygen—causes a general strain on the body. We point this out because it can be prevented and the resulting troubles can be avoided. The woman suffers if they are allowed to accumulate.

Among these troubles are those of the venous circulation. As a rule, we merely note them, believing that we can do little to relieve them. Now, without pretending to work miracles, we very often manage to prevent the appearance of these circulatory troubles, or to prevent them getting worse once they have appeared. We shall see how.

Let us explain the 'venous circulation'. We are concerned only with the part of the body below the heart, and in particular with the legs and pelvis. When the blood, which comes from the heart and circulates in the arteries, has been distributed into the fine capillaries, its pressure becomes extremely weak. It is then collected in the venous plexus. A question then arises: how does the blood manage to return to the heart? It must go up, since we live standing up half the time. It can do so for several reasons:

1. It uses what is left of the pressure, little as this is.

2. The venous tissues are very supple and covered with tiny muscles.

3. The veins of the legs are provided with valves, rather like

small cups, which let the blood go through, but, when they close, prevent it from going back.

4. This allows advantage to be taken of: (*a*) the arterial circulation of which the pulse wave is transmitted to the veins and pushes the blood very slightly, and (*b*) the active movements of the individual, and especially the contractions of the muscles.

The human venous circulation is very delicate, and must be neither clogged nor obstructed. We understand why so many people say, 'My legs are heavy' or 'I have pains in my legs,' and we also understand the formation of varicose veins and the troubles which follow. Now can we help the pregnant woman?

The uterus and its contents occupy the abdominal cavity. It takes up room there at the expense of all the other organs which, remember, continue to function. (The woman who is expecting a baby tends to forget this.) The organs are pushed back and compressed. Some of them stand this very well; others not so well.

This applies to two large veins which, having collected the blood from the legs, pour it into another still larger vein. These two iliac veins, found in the pelvis, are compressed by the uterus. There is a more or less pronounced slowing of the circulation when they enter the main vein (inferior vena cava). Consequently the blood in the leg veins is held up.

There is no need to dwell on the troubles which result. Once more, it is better to see how we can prevent these troubles.

1. We cannot in practice influence the pressure of the blood in the veins.

2. It is possible to maintain the elasticity of the tissues of the veins.

3. Above all we can try to maintain as much as possible the valvular structure of the veins, by the use of active movements, that is to say muscular contractions:

(*a*) at the junction of the iliac veins by the use of the muscles of the pelvis,

(*b*) in the legs by the use of all their muscles,

(*c*) and in the feet by the use of the plantar muscles.

Movements of the foot entail active working of the muscles of the sole, which for this reason is considered to be the most important starting point of the venous return from the legs. It is a grave and yet very common mistake to consider flattening of the arch—what we call flat foot—only from an aesthetic angle. The flattening of the plantar arch deprives the foot of its mobility and, at the same time, of its function in propelling the blood.

So you must not be surprised when we insist upon exercises for the feet and legs. In the pregnant woman the ligaments soften, and the joints become looser and more supple. This is all right for the ligaments and joints of the pelvis. For the ligaments and joints of the foot it is not all right.

The exercises taught in the first lecture must be fully carried out. You should gradually increase the time devoted to them.

There is one frequent mistake. To strengthen the abdominal muscles, the following exercises are often used:

1. Lying on the back, lift both legs together to the vertical position, then slowly lower them.

2. Lying on the back, the two feet fixed under something—say a chest of drawers—raise the trunk slowly; then let it fall back slowly.

These two exercises must be forbidden. They are harmful and can even be dangerous in pregnancy. They require very powerful contractions of the muscles attached to the femur and the pelvis on the one side, and to the lumbar vertebrae on the other. While contracting—and they contract strongly—they pull the vertebral column forwards and downwards, thus increasing the lumbar curve. This is easily proved by sliding your hand between the back and the surface on which you are lying. When you are at rest, your hand is held between your back and the surface; as soon as the legs rise, your hand is freed.

We are now going over to the practical work to see what you have learnt to do since the last lecture.

Lecture 4

The Principles of the Method

WE are going to begin this lecture with a journey into the past. When you were twelve and an attentive pupil, you probably began to delve into the mysteries of the reproduction of plants. It was a marvellous thing, a real fairy tale, this adventure of a seed becoming a plant. Your teacher explained that if a seed of any kind were placed in the soil, it would burst open in the earth, force its way through, and, one day, would appear in the form of a little plant. It was green. Spring was here, and then it grew and grew and grew to form a strong stem. Using corn as an example, they told you that it would produce a magnificent ear, and, if we took all the grains contained in the ear and resowed them next season, the process would be repeated.

This made you interested in the phenomenon of reproduction in general, but, during that year, only the reproduction of plants was explained. Nothing was said about animals. Nothing was said about human beings. But when you reached fourteen, you were probably taught how animals reproduce. Generally at school the story of animal reproduction is treated briefly. You are told that certain species reproduce directly. That means they come into the world in their final form but smaller—for example the dog, the cat and the rabbit. You are told these are viviparous. You had to remember this name—it would be useful for composition—but afterwards you forgot it.

Then you were given examples of animals which do not reproduce directly. The hen lays an egg and sits on it; it breaks open and a little chick emerges to become a hen or a cock, and so on. These animals, you were told, are oviparous. No doubt you were given examples of animals passing through many more stages. But that was all. You were told nothing about human reproduction. At present in French schools there is no official instruction about the most important event in our existence—transmitting and creating life. But although at school

58

you were told nothing about the reproduction of human beings, did you not try to find out? Yes, of course! We all tried to get details, and as soon as we could. One day, probably at school, a senior girl destroyed the last of your illusions about the magic power of the stork. Of course, it was a wonderful story, but the older girl laughed. She said: 'The stork, you don't believe that! Babies grow in women's stomachs!' What an eye-opener! A baby growing in the stomach of a woman? 'One day I shall be a woman.'

The girl explained some more and you took your new ideas in and immediately thought: 'And when I have a baby, it will grow in my stomach.' The older girl added: 'I will show you when we are outside.' And as it happened, shortly afterwards, you met a woman well on in her pregnancy, say eight months. At eight months, it is obvious, and seems all the bigger to the young girl, because she is shorter, and she sees it from below. You stopped, surprised, and said to the older girl: 'A baby in the stomach? Yes, but how does it come out?' The question may sound odd, but in reality it is very serious. That day, you first realized the marked disproportion between the size of the baby and the possible ways for it to come out. This matter of disproportion caused a mental conflict in you. It was the first shock, and a very great one, to which others would be added later. Indeed, every time you brought up the subject of pregnancy, read or heard accounts of it, you always came back to the same question, and always got no answer—at least not a reasonable answer.

Later, perhaps, you saw pregnancy close to. A person you knew, or a relative, had a child. You learned what happened at her confinement —that during labour she screamed. Screamed! So she was in pain. You also learned that she lost blood; but, as she lost blood, it was dangerous! You notice that, for the first days after the confinement, she stayed in bed and the doctor and midwife came to see her several times. Therefore, it was a disease. And from that moment, in your impressionable young girl's mind, confinement was associated with the ideas of pain and danger. And every time that you talked or read about confinements, the event was associated with these two ideas.

But you were not going to remain a young girl for ever. You would get married one day, and then. . . . And then, here you are—which means that this time it is not a neighbour or a relative who is expecting the day. It is *you*.

In the past, when women discovered that they were going to have a baby, what did they think of? They naturally thought about the end of the pregnancy, which meant a time of pain and danger. They did not think about it with much pleasure and quite often they were afraid. A woman may feel so much fear, apprehension and dread that she makes her husband share them. They talk about the coming event, the end of the pregnancy, the confinement. The husband sees it all from a different angle, 'It's only the beginning,' he says to himself. 'If it's like this now, what will it be like at the end?' He reprimands her. 'You still have seven or eight months to go. So don't worry. Everything generally goes all right.' These simple words reveal doubts which confirm her own. She may also talk to her mother. After all, she has usually confided in her. One day, she tells her that she is going to be a grand-mother. This makes the mother feel a bit older, but after all that is beside the point. She is very moved, and how does she react? Usually, she says: 'You're going to have a baby. . . . Oh! my poor little thing!' But the mother does not stop there. She begins to talk about her own confinement—the girl's birth, with all the details. How it began, how it went on, the increasing pain, what happened at the clinic—nothing is left out. The moral of the story is that to have a baby you must suffer. 'You know, my poor dear, you must go through it. It can't be helped. It's part of the confinement. It's normal. That's what will happen. . . .'

The mother repeats: 'Of course, you'll have pain, but when it's all over, you'll laugh over it.' Then, not wanting to leave the girl with these unpleasant thoughts, she may add: 'Yes, but I know you'll be brave and, besides, we'll be there. We'll help you.' The girl does not know how, mark you, but they will be there! Outside the family circle a woman, during her pregnancy, is bound to hear some story of confinement; and then, of course, it has to be a difficult one, with nothing left out. It gives her a shock; and the shocks add up and affect her nervous system.

Now the physiologist, Pavlov, worked all his life to show how the nervous system acts and how the environment influences the individual. Pavlov discovered that the brain was the great regulator of the nervous system and that our organic and functional equilibria depend on it.

We have just seen that, although officially schoolchildren were given no lessons on human reproduction, they all tried to find out the secret details. We call this curiosity. In more scientific terms, we say that it is the absolute reflex of investigation. Now each individual, when he comes into the world, can respond to certain needs or demands which arise as soon as he finds himself in the environment where he must live. This ability to react is called an *absolute reflex*.

We do not learn these inborn reflexes; they exist at birth and we keep them all our life. They form the material basis of our adaptation to our environment.

Without them survival would not be possible. Is it not essential to be able to eat, sleep, accept what is useful, reject what is harmful, to run away from or avoid what is dangerous? But it is clear that, if these reflexes, and hence the behaviour which reflects them, were to remain only thus rudimentary, our life would be entirely vegetable, and not very exciting. We should be among the lower animals.

Very quickly these inborn reflexes, which are the result of permanent nervous connexions between a definite unchanging stimulus—hunger for example—and a specific act of the organism, eating, will serve as a basis for the formation of another category of reflexes which are more delicate, precise and subtle. Thanks to these new reflexes, the individual will be able to respond and adapt in a definite way to the changing conditions of the external environment. The sum of the reflexes acquired by an individual in the course of his life may be called his upbringing.

Let us try to give a simple example.

1. At birth, a baby sucks without having learnt how to do it. This is an inborn reflex.

2. He cries when he is hungry. This is also an inborn reflex.

3. He cries if, when taken out of his cradle, he is not fed straight away. It is the change of position which conditions his cries and demands.

He may cry when he sees his mother if she waits too long before feeding him. It is the sight of the person which now conditions his cries.

These two last examples show that the change of position or the sight of his mother is the *direct signal* of feeding.

4. Later, the infant will cry at the sound of his mother's voice, at feeding time. The words are now the *indirect signal* of feeding.

This example shows that words are substituted very early for a direct stimulus.

Let us take some more examples. You know that it is not necessary to burn a child to make him understand that fire is dangerous. Nor is it necessary to throw a baby out of the window to make him understand that a fall is dangerous. It is enough to explain it in words. In short, everything around us has an effect upon us, and words can replace any direct stimulus.

It was Pavlov who gave the name 'stimuli' to all the information which reaches us, both from the external and our own internal environment. These stimuli act first on the sensory organs (receptors), which transmit them through the nervous system to the brain, which receives, analyses, then regroups and synthesizes all the information and reacts to it. Finally, it is the brain which co-ordinates and directs all our activities.

But let us examine, to illustrate all this, what actually happens in our own bodies. You are in good health and alert. All the organs in your body are working. But do you feel these organs working when you are well and fully conscious? Obviously not. This does not mean that your organs are not sensitive. Actually from each of them stimuli are constantly arising. They start from the little nerve endings which are found in their walls. They pass along the nervous pathways to the brain, to which they give information about the functions of the organs. But when we are in good health and fully conscious, these stimuli, on reaching the brain, are stopped. They meet a barrier they cannot cross, because they are not strong enough. It is said that the brain possesses a braking power; it owes this to the fact that it has greater strength than the stimuli. We can say that the currents resulting from the stimulation of the nerve endings in the internal organs are under 5 or 8 volts—while that of the brain is 20 or 30 volts. The stimuli are too weak to cross the brain's threshold of sensation.

Yet an individual in perfect health can, in certain circumstances, feel his internal organs in an unpleasant and even painful way. This may result from a strong emotion. During your life, you have experienced upsetting events such as receiving a telegram which brings bad news. At such moments you feel dizzy or sick; your heart beats strongly and quickly. Yet these troubles are not caused by a lesion in the organs. Why, then, do we feel them?

The brain's threshold of sensation is suddenly lowered. Let us return to electricity. We can say that there was a short-circuit; a great fall in voltage has removed the brain's braking power. As a result, it is in an inferior condition and allows these same stimuli to pass through in disorder.

We have chosen an example of a sudden fall in the brain's threshold of sensation. But the phenomenon can also occur slowly, after a long succession of weak shocks. Although the effect of these shocks on the nervous system is not sudden, it is sure and equally harmful.

To summarize:

1. The stimuli from internal organs are weaker than the brain's force and do not pass through.

2. Sometimes the normal stimuli from our internal organs cross the threshold of sensation. This happens when external stimuli have had a bad effect on the brain, lowering its threshold.

But inversely external stimuli can help the brain; they can maintain or raise its threshold. With the brain at a good tension, normal but stronger stimuli can be transmitted from the internal organs, but they will not cross the threshold of sensation.

Let us reconsider the conditions in which you have lived since childhood. The successive shocks of which we have spoken have resulted in a slow disorganization of your nervous system and its equilibrium.

During pregnancy the woman waits for the pains. She dreads them more and more as term approaches. At the same time, the strength of her brain threshold diminishes. The first regular contractions marking the onset of labour, though of normal strength, create an emotional shock which finally upsets her nervous equilibrium. These contractions then have enough strength to cross the threshold of sensation. They have assumed the character of a pain signal. They were in effect accompanied by pains.

We must now consider the attitude of the medical profession. They can be gauged by the progress of a confinement. The woman is probably greeted at the maternity hospital by a midwife or a nurse—very nicely—with 'Good morning, dear.' Why 'dear'? Because the word is very protective. You are taken under her wing; you are a poor woman who is going to suffer. You will not be called 'dear' by us but 'Mrs. So-and-So', like everybody else, because you do not need protection any more.

In the past, you were immediately asked a serious question, 'When did your pains start, dear?' You replied and they noted it: 'The pains started at such and such a time.' The second question was: 'How often are the pains coming?' You answered, and it was taken down: 'They are coming every ten or twelve minutes.' Then they added: 'Not oftener? They're not very close together. You're only just beginning. It isn't too painful yet, is it?' This question meant: 'It's nothing now, but soon you will see. . . .'

Then there was the first examination in the ward. Usually, you were among other women in labour. You could see or hear them, and it was a series of shocks. The doctors regarded the pain as a normal feature, a condition of labour.

Confinement was considered by everybody as a passive event, a sort of condition or disease for which nobody could do anything. The woman remained inactive, and her behaviour was the reflection of all these beliefs. This attitude was wrong. The woman should not just wait during confinement.

We must revise all our ideas. We must work together. All of us must learn. When we understand, we perform well. And, thanks to our preparation, pregnancy and childbirth become active events.

The woman can follow the progress of her pregnancy and analyse certain physiological features—for example the movements of her baby. From a certain period she will also be able to analyse the contractions of the uterus and carry out certain exercises. She must try to understand what she is doing, the reason for the work and its effect on her confinement. The medical people look after her and also instruct and guide her.

At the time of childbirth, the woman will put all she has learnt into practice. As soon as labour begins—and she will know how it begins—she will observe, analyse, control and discover the value of her training. In directing her labour, she will make it shorter. The aim of her activity will be to respond to the organic processes occurring at different times in labour. She will consciously take part in the event. She will no longer submit to it; she will adapt to it.

We try to make you feel part of your confinement, and not to distract you from it—not make you feel separate from the contractions, for example. This would be absurd. And the rôle of the medical attendants will consist not only of keeping an eye on the progress of your confinement but telling you how it is getting on. If you do not know, how can you act appropriately? But you, too, must tell the doctors. Their observations and yours can be compared, and labour will be conducted better.

Finally, the rôle of the medical attendants will be to improve your performance if necessary. You are not infallible. You can forget. You can make mistakes. The doctor, as well as making clinical observations, will concentrate on using the right words; because, as you are aware, words have a great influence on the behaviour of the individual.

You no longer start your confinement, as women used to do,

resigned to pain accepted as a necessity. The knowledge you acquire will increase your state of awareness; and you will put the rules and ideas you have been taught into practice. You will experience child-birth from beginning to end, remaining fully conscious, and you will thus emerge triumphant from the most wonderful battle of your existence—that of creating life.

But before coming to the end of this lecture, I should like to give you some very important advice. Very often, women have an un-fortunate tendency to think that, thanks to the training, their confine-ment will be very simple. This is a great mistake. Actually, childbirth without pain—and this I have repeated for more than four years—is not childbirth without effort. The result you obtain will depend upon how you make use of what you have learned. This knowledge is both theoretical and practical, the two sides being always closely linked. Never separate the practical side from the underlying theory. Do not separate, either, theory from practice.

Professor Paul Langevin has said: 'Theory results from action and creates it.'

Lecture 5

Respiration

ODAY, we are going to talk about respiration in relation to
pregnancy and childbirth.

The volume of air breathed in and out by an individual in
normal conditions is very small—about one litre. Every time you
breathe in, you take in a litre of air, and you breathe out about the same
amount. A litre is really very little. But the capacity of the lungs is much
greater. Have you any idea of the average lung capacity of a woman,
for example? Between three and three and a half litres. So that, after
breathing in and out, at the end of expiration, there is still some air
in the lungs. This air is well mixed and we divide it arbitrarily into
two parts. The first is called complementary air, which we can expel
by using certain muscles; we shall see which shortly. The second is
called residual air, which we cannot affect.

Let us now go into the mechanism of respiration. We can then
explain quite a lot of things related to pregnancy and childbirth.

Breathing is essentially the result of the work of a muscle which is
well known to you—the diaphragm. This muscle does not act directly
on the lungs, but through certain bones—the thoracic cage. There is
thus a series of actions. A muscle, the diaphragm, acts on the bones of
the thoracic cage, which then act on the lungs. It is essential to keep
this in mind; otherwise you will not be able to understand how the
diaphragm works.

The diaphragm is widely attached to the inner sides of the last or
lower ribs; very widely all round the thoracic cage, and, at the back,
to the vertebral column, where, however, it is not attached directly.
It is shaped like the quarter of a sphere, which means that from back to
front, from the vertebral column to the front of the chest, it is convex.
It is also attached all around the thoracic cage. The diaphragm seen
from the front would diagrammatically have this convex shape. I
will not try to describe how deep it is; it does not matter.

66

Now here is the vertebral column. It is at the back, rising here and going down there. Here are the lungs, immediately above the diaphragm. The diaphragm is shown here at the end of expiration, after a complete respiratory cycle. I am going to try now to show it at the end of inspiration, when you have taken air into the lungs. At this moment, its shape changes completely. In inspiration, contrary to what you might think, it does not rise; it falls. At the same time, it flattens, spreads out, and tends to rise at the edges. Here it is during inspiration. I repeat: at its edges, it is raised. Then, all that part of the thoracic cage, which it took up before, is freed.

Of course, from this diagram it is difficult to understand how, when the diaphragm falls and gives up this space, it can allow the lungs to fill with air. Why? Because the thoracic cage is not shown here. Now I have told you that the diaphragm acts through the thoracic cage. But if I were to try to show the thoracic cage on the diagram, it would be difficult both to explain and to understand. So I will make a comparison, a very simple one—an umbrella. Here is a closed umbrella. When it is closed we will compare it with expiration, when the lungs are relatively empty. Now we are going to open the umbrella; and say that this is inspiration. You understand: closed, it is expiration; open, inspiration. But why? Consider the mechanism of the umbrella. For it to open, all the ribs which move the cover must have a point of support and this is the shaft.

Let us consider the problem now in terms of the human body. What support does the diaphragm find in our body in order to extend the thoracic cage? This support is made up of all the organs situated immediately below it—the abdominal contents. The contents are kept in position by the abdominal muscles; limited at the back by the vertebral column, and below by the pelvis. In the first phase of inspiration, the central part of the diaphragm (the phrenic part), as it falls, is supported by, and settles down on to, the abdominal contents. Simultaneously, or nearly, the muscle fibres coming from the central part start working and act on the ribs which have remained free. They transmit quite complicated movements to the ribs. With each inspiration, the ribs turn, rise, move forward and spread out, all at the same time. These movements are made possible by the way in which the different axes of the ribs are orientated, and especially by the way they articulate at the back with the thoracic vertebrae.

Following the three movements described, the thoracic cage has expanded in three directions—vertically, when the diaphragm falls;

from front to back when the ribs come forward; and also from side to side when the ribs spread out. Among these movements, there is one which interests you much more than the others—the lowering of the diaphragm, which must rest on the abdominal contents. Your abdomen at this time contains a baby which is growing and developing. The volume of the uterus has increased so much that it now comes into contact, indirect of course, with the diaphragm, through its upper part which is called the fundus. From about the sixth month, the fundus of the uterus serves as a point of support for the diaphgram at each inspiration.

It is not enough to know the theory of this relationship; you must become aware of its physical reality. You can do this through a breath-

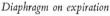
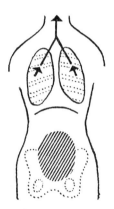
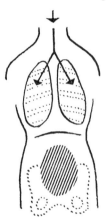

Diaphragm on expiration   *Diaphragm on inspiration*

ing exercise which you will learn at the end of the lecture. This exercise will require some attention. Never carry out any of these exercises mechanically or automatically.

The lowering of the diaphragm and its support by the fundus of the uterus are advantageous, and you will gain from them during delivery. On the other hand, the compression raises a slight difficulty which you will have to remedy during dilatation.

The diaphragm is the essential muscle of respiration. But, during inspiration, it does not work alone. It is helped by other muscles; and some of these, the auxiliary muscles of inspiration, you can control. It is precisely these that we ask you not to use when you carry out the exercise which you will shortly be taught. You must leave most of the work to the diaphragm, which will thus become stronger more quickly; besides, in using it by itself, you will understand better and sooner how it works, what it can do and what its limitations are. Then you will be able to use it in a logical way.

You know the muscles not to be used, since you used them a lot at school. You remember you did gymnastics? In the playground, you were drawn up in lines and told to do exercises, which included breathing movements. They stood you on tip-toe. You breathed in, raising your arms; then you breathed out, lowering your arms. It was very good, well co-ordinated. You were made to raise your arms simply because this movement allowed these muscles to work properly. During your breathing exercises, you must do exactly the opposite. That is to say:

> always keep your arms alongside your body, relaxed;
> hold the shoulders low;
> turn the palms to face backwards.

You now know the most important things about the mechanism of inspiration.

As for expiration, it is simplicity itself. When the diaphragm has finished its work, it relaxes. The thoracic cage is no longer held in extension and it falls back. It obeys the law of gravity. Expiration is a passive process; there is no voluntary or involuntary activity apart from the tone of certain muscles. During expiration air is expelled freely from our lungs, until the moment when the pressure of the air remaining in the lungs becomes the same as that of the external air. Of course, when the pressures become equal, expiration stops and a new inspiration begins. The diaphragm contracts, the thoracic cage extends, you breathe in; the diaphragm again stops working, the thoracic cage falls back and so on. Clearly, what I have just described concerns the ordinary habitual breathing you are using now.

But when the pressures are equal, as I told you at the beginning, there is still some air in the lungs. And I also told you that it was possible to expel this complementary air. We then talked about muscles which allowed us to do this. Now we are going to learn the second important relationship which exists between respiration, pregnancy and childbirth. It is remarkable. The muscles which expel the complementary air from your lungs are those which enable you during delivery to help the uterus to empty its contents—to expel the baby. They are the abdominal muscles. I repeat, the abdominal muscles in the woman are expiratory, and at childbirth they take part in delivery.

Your abdominal muscles are attached above to the lowest ribs; nearly the same as those to which the diaphragm is attached. From those lowest ribs, the abdominal muscles pass to the pelvis. Here they become attached very extensively to the iliac crests and the iliac spines; furthermore, to the sides and the lowest part of the pelvis and also to the most forward part—the pubis. I advise you to remember this name, the pubis. We shall talk about it quite often; it is sometimes called the 'pubic symphysis'.

Let us summarize: lowest ribs, pelvis, pubis in front. When the pelvis is immobilized—and it is immobilized when you are sitting or lying, your legs more or less extended—the abdominal muscles contract. The fixed point is below, in the pelvis, and their contraction will affect the parts remaining free—that is to say, the upper part, the ribs. There is a strong pull which corresponds to a force exerted vertically from above downwards which will transmit movements to the ribs—movements exactly opposite to those described above, which means that the thoracic cage will become smaller and smaller; and, in becoming smaller in this way, it will compress the lungs, from which the air will be forcibly expelled. These abdominal muscles take their turn and finish the work begun by the diaphragm.

Action of the abdominal muscles

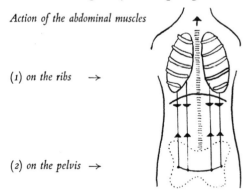

(1) on the ribs →

(2) on the pelvis →

And now we will summarize the two important phases of respiration, exactly as you will have to practise them during the exercises.

During the inspiration you will take in a large quantity of air and also make the diaphragm work more strongly. And it will become stronger. By learning how to make it work, you will be able later on to control it much better.

During expiration, you will expel the complementary air. But this complementary air is composed almost entirely of CO_2 (a gas which cannot produce energy or maintain life); and what will replace this CO_2? A quantity of fresh air containing more O_2 so that, during the exercise, the absorption of O_2 will be much greater. But during the exercise only; you must not overdo it. I will tell you how much to do shortly. So, temporarily, you get more oxygen. This will have a good effect on your present condition. From now on you will have to do a somewhat different exercise as well as those which you began several weeks ago. But is what is true during pregnancy also true during childbirth? Even more true, since you will have a lot of work to do, using up a deal of energy, requiring plenty of oxygen. Thus, once more, through good training, you will be able to meet and satisfy these needs.

Here is a most important point. Your abdominal muscles work when you expel the complementary air; they work hard, therefore they will become stronger. You will see the difference between now and the day of childbirth, and you will realize that you have got a stronger abdominal wall. You will have learned little by little to make these muscles work. At delivery, your efforts will be much more effective thanks to a stronger abdominal wall, and *especially* because you will be able to control the work of these muscles. Now, contrary to what was previously thought, the effect of an expulsive effort depends much more on the way the woman controls it than on its strength. You are going to learn all this gradually through your exercises—the one you have to do from now on, as well as others to be added later.

Delivery is regarded as a time when the baby may be injured. As soon as delivery begins, the baby leaves the uterus, and enters a narrow canal, limited by a bone, the pelvis, that it must cross by force. Delivery must not take long. The best way available up to now to make it quick is the one you have been taught today. (We have been trying to find a way for a long time and we are still trying.) To have to revive the baby at birth was common in the past, but is exceptional today. The woman in labour works not only for herself but even more for her baby. He uses up large quantities of oxygen during delivery, and his needs have to be satisfied by his mother.

Let us now come to the breathing exercise. It is very simple, but it should be done very carefully.

1. Breathe in deeply, preferably through your nose.

2. Breathe out in two phases: first phase, passive. You open your mouth, and let the air come out from your lungs as you do when breathing normally, except that, instead of doing it through the nose,

you will do it through your mouth. You will expel a little more air, because you took in more. So the first phase is passive; the air comes out freely until the pressures are equal. Then, instead of breathing in again— you will feel the need to do this—you must instead voluntarily expel the complementary air. This is the active phase of expiration. To make your abdominal muscles work properly, this is how you will do it:

Imagine a lighted candle placed about twenty inches in front of you. All you have to do is blow the flame so that it is disturbed but not put out. Why such detail? Because the flame of a candle placed at this distance is a very small objective; and, if you want to reach it by blowing, you must take careful aim. And to take aim, you must put your lips together. In this way you make an obstacle to the air that you have to expel. A certain force is necessary to overcome this obstacle. Keep it up for a definite length of time: long enough to expel the complementary air from your lungs. This will make your abdominal muscles work at a certain strength for a definite time.

If we had said to you, 'Here is a candle, at such and such a distance. You must blow it out,' you would have taken a lot of air into your lungs; you would have puffed it out very quickly, and you would certainly have blown the candle out. Your abdominal muscles would most certainly have worked, but you could not have found out properly how they work, because it would have been done too quickly. This is why I mention all these details. You must do this exercise three times a day—say in the morning, at noon before lunch, and in the evening. The women still at work should do it twice daily—morning and evening, say, if you do not come home for lunch. But, as soon as you stop working, do it three times a day. So, as a rule, three times a day, and each time three to five minutes.

Begin with five minutes, but, if you feel tired, be satisfied with four minutes. If you are still tired, reduce to three minutes; three minutes is always sufficient. After the exercise you should not feel stiff. To avoid this, especially in the abdominal muscles, you must not overdo it and not try to breathe in and blow out too deeply. Do not forget that, although they must tone up your muscles, the aim of these exercises is not to make you an athlete. However, if you do feel a bit stiff, do not worry. It is not very important and will quickly go. You should not get dizzy either during the exercises: if you feel the least bit giddy, it is because you breathe too quickly, which means that you must limit the number of respirations. One respiration consists of one inspiration plus one expiration.

The rate of respiration in the pregnant woman is noticeably in-creased—fifteen to twenty per minute. You have new needs to satisfy. When you do your exercise, the respiration falls, according to the woman, to between three to nine. It depends on the lung capacity of the individual, and also her needs. Try nine a minute, and, if you get the least bit dizzy, try less.

You will do this exercise usually lying down, sometimes sitting, and preferably without a belt or brassière. Do it in the morning, when you are still in bed, and at night, when you are going to bed. The best position is like that in a low deck chair. The thighs are at a slight angle to what you are lying on (as a rule the bed) and the calves are supported at a level between that of the head and the pelvis.

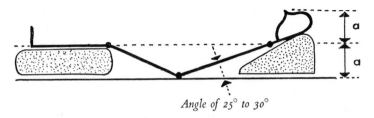

Angle of 25° to 30°

Also it will be better if your back is kept fairly straight. Support yourself if necessary with pillows and cushions.

I am going to describe the physical sensations which accompany this exercise. We are coming to the practical side of the lecture. Do not expect, however, these sensations to occur exactly when you begin to do it, today or tomorrow. Through them you will be able to discover, observe and understand all the relationships between respiration and pregnancy and childbirth. But you may feel the sensations clearly only after you have done the exercise for five or six days. Some women need four to five days, others seven to eight, and still others, ten or fifteen. That depends on your reactions. So do not be surprised if at first you hardly feel anything.

In inspiration, your diaphragm falls and presses on the fundus of the uterus. You will feel this pressure in the region of the pit of your stomach as a rough indication. The pressure does not involve the outside at all; it is inside—just a bit behind the stomach. The sensation of pressure spreads out downwards and a little to the left and to the right. It is this that you will have to observe during inspiration.

During the passive phase of expiration, the diaphragm rises and as a result frees the abdominal contents. The only real sensation is that your abdomen will become relatively soft again in the region of the stomach. During the active phase of expiration, when you begin to blow at the candle, you will have a lot of things to notice. The first thing is the pull exerted by your abdominal muscles, not on the last ribs, but immediately below them. Another pull will also be exerted below in the region of the pubis. Do not forget where the abdominal muscles are attached; above to the lowest ribs, below to the pelvis, in front to the pubis. You will feel a pull in the region of the pubis, which will spread out to the right and left towards the groins. But it is mainly the second sensation that I am going to stress. Try to notice carefully the pressure which your abdominal muscles exert on the sides of your uterus. When the abdominal muscles contract, they strongly compress the uterus.

You should discriminate between two forms of compression. One is exerted from the sides, the work of the abdominal muscles on the uterus; the other from above, the work of the diaphragm on the fundus of the uterus. Why must you try to differentiate between them? Because you have to use these two groups of muscles during delivery; and you cannot use them properly unless you have tried to understand, before your confinement, how they work, how strong they are and in what direction they work. Only then will you make proper use of them during childbirth.

The third sensation you must notice is the tilting of the pelvis. Perhaps you have noticed it already. Remember, the abdominal muscles pull the pelvis upwards. You do not clearly feel this movement of the pelvis in the pelvis itself; but you know that the pelvis has tilted because your vertebral column is straightened out; and being straightened out, it will press strongly on the bed, that is, on the surface on which you do your exercises.

And now we are going on to the exercise. I am going to demonstrate it, and afterwards you must observe all the physical sensations described. The exercise is done first in the sitting position, but at home you will do it lying down. I add that from time to time you should exercise sitting down. This is because, during your confinement, you will not be lying down all the time. Try to exercise in all possible positions.

We are going to start with a completely mechanical exercise, a trial which will probably convince you. Then we will analyse the sensations which have been described.

You noticed that the baby moved during or immediately after the exercise.

We are going to take the opportunity of mentioning two particularly interesting things which normally accompany every pregnancy.

At about the fourth month, the woman begins to feel the movements of the baby. She notices that they are very irregular and may come at any time. They happen at unexpected moments under any conditions. Yet we shall see that they do have 'favourite' times.

Women can detect the place where the movement occurs very accurately, even though it may last such a short time. The place is not always the same, though here again there may be a 'favourite spot'. Women usually say, 'He is kicking me.'

Women react to these movements differently. Some say, 'It's nice,' others, 'It's a nuisance.' In any case we shall benefit from them if we pay careful attention to them. By relating the uterus to the movements, you can learn the position of the uterus in the abdomen and become familiar with this muscle.

You must take all possible advantage of the time when the baby moves, which is mainly when you yourself move, and also during the breathing exercises.

We confirm what we said in the last lecture. We must realize the relationships which exist between the organs directly or indirectly involved in parturition.

Lecture 6

Neuromuscular Training

I N the last lecture we talked about the movements of the baby during pregnancy. You had to define his position in your abdomen. Today, we shall talk of the contractions of the uterus during pregnancy, so that you will know what they mean physically.

These contractions can very well pass unnoticed. You may scarcely be aware that they exist; or you may feel them very faintly. But I will give you a few details, and you will all be able to recognize them.

The contractions of the uterus and the movements of the baby are often superimposed. Both are irregular, and you cannot predict at what moment a contraction is going to occur. However, you will be able to differentiate it from the movements. Women say that from time to time during the day they feel—and it is not only a feeling— that their abdomen hardens and protrudes. However, if some of you have not felt it, do not be surprised.

I have told you how to analyse the movements of the baby. Now I am going to tell you how to analyse the contractions. These occur particularly when the woman moves, for example, from sitting to standing or vice versa; or, still more clearly, when going to bed or getting up. But the best time for the woman to find out what they are like is when she goes to bed. Tonight, in bed, you will feel your abdomen carefully and you will notice—you must have noticed it already—that one side remains soft and the other hard. After a certain time the side which is soft becomes hard. This is a contraction. This hardening will be felt through the abdominal wall; so you will try at the same time not to contract your abdominal muscles, but keep them soft.

Naturally, the first time you feel the uterus harden through the abdominal wall you will not be able to analyse it adequately. But you will feel it again and observe it many times, so that you will eventually know—and this is precisely what we are asking you—that the contraction begins above the pubis. You will notice that it spreads towards the groins and involves the whole of the uterus (it does not involve just one point at one place), while it becomes stronger, reaches its peak, stays there a few moments, then begins to weaken, further decreases and finally disappears. All this takes half to one minute. What you have to do therefore during pregnancy is to learn the essential process of childbirth, so that, as soon as childbirth starts, you recognize it and do the right things. You adapt to the contraction instead of submitting to it as women used to do. In brief, when you arrive at the maternity home to give birth to your baby, you will not find yourself at a loss; you will put to use the knowledge you have acquired.

So do not neglect to observe the movements of the baby and the contractions of the uterus.

But since we have come to this subject, I am going to tell you at once the difference between a contraction during pregnancy and a contraction in childbirth. It is very simple. At present, your contractions are irregular. During childbirth, they become regular; also they will become stronger, and above all, will alter in type.

Now we are going to talk about neuromuscular training. I do not mean simple muscular relaxation and, even less, relaxation. Relaxation is only one side of the question, a result obtained from neuromuscular training. In the second lecture I talked at some length of two groups of muscles— the diaphragm and the abdominal muscles—so that you know theoretically exactly where these muscles are situated in your body, which parts of the bones they are attached to or inserted into, and finally what movements these muscles can impart to these bones when they contract. But, while you know the theory of all these things, you must also have begun to appreciate their physical reality, since, at the end of the lecture, you were taught an exercise to act as a link between what you were taught theoretically and what must become evident to you physically. Why have you been able to realize where these muscles are in your body? Why do you know how these muscles work, how strongly and in what direction they work?

Because there is a nervous process by which you become aware of them. It is very simple. Each time you contract a muscle, an order first leaves your brain; there is, if you like, in the brain a centre of excitation which starts to work. This excitation, this order, this motor command, is sent through nervous pathways to a muscle or group of muscles, and this responds by contracting. The excitation is then passed to other, very numerous, nerve endings, contained in the muscle. All these nerve endings join up, forming one nerve which connects with the brain. When the excitation returns, it is transformed into sensation.

Our brain possesses, in fact, sensory centres which make this process possible. You can become conscious of your muscles, know exactly where they are, how they work and what their work is. The brain—and this is what we are trying to bring out—is the centre of our sensations. But the muscle can very well become sensitive; it can be felt without contracting. For this it must be stimulated from the exterior either by the individual or by somebody else. If, for example, I prick you, or pinch you, you would feel the muscle concerned. It is in a state of rest—and you feel it without its becoming active. So there are two possibilities, internal and external excitation.

And if neither excitation occurs, are our muscles sensitive? Not especially; at this moment, the muscles of the forearms are in a state of rest, your forearms rest on your thighs. Do you feel your back muscles now? Not especially. I do not mean by this that the individual has no idea of the position of his body in space. In fact he has a very precise idea, but this is due to another phenomenon. You do not feel the muscles of your back. They must contract for you to feel them. If, for instance, you drop your head you immediately feel the muscles of your back.

Let us return to the example of the forearm. My right forearm now rests on the table, and the muscles which act on this forearm are not working. Consider the biceps—everybody knows this muscle; the biceps is one of the flexors of the forearm on the upper arm. I know it is there but, as it does not work, I do not feel it, at least not particularly. I am now going to contract it; I make this movement—flexion of the forearm on the upper arm. My biceps took part in the movement. An order left the brain, my biceps contracted and I felt it. If you wish, we will say that the work of my brain is expressed as motor activity. Now I am going to let my forearm return to the table very gently. My biceps is still working. but it is used now to restrain the fall of my forearm on the table. It restrains its fall because the strength of the current sent to it has been reduced.

Let us make a comparison; imagine that you are listening to the radio. When you want it to be very loud you increase the current; if you want to turn it down you reduce the current. I repeat this flexion of the forearm on the upper arm. My brain has worked again; an order has been given: my biceps reacted and so on. The activity of my brain is once more translated into movement. Something different happens if I let my arm fall back on the table. Instead of taking the example of the radio, we will take a much simpler example, that of an electric light. Suppose that the light is on. To turn it off, I am going to use the switch and suddenly cut off the current. And if, in my brain, I cut off the current which is being sent at this moment to my biceps, what will happen? The biceps completely stops working, and my forearm, no longer held up, falls heavily. We say then that motor activity is inhibited. The excitation of the active motor centres has stopped. Other processes have started to work and have acted on the first. It is the brain which has ordered the muscular work to stop.

Muscular relaxation corresponds to this phenomenon in the nervous system. I have pointed out that, when my biceps was contracting, it corresponded to cerebral activity converted into motor activity. But when my biceps no longer worked, did my brain work? Of course! Except that in this second case, its activity resulted in stopping the motor activity.

In both cases, the brain is working, which means that muscular relaxation corresponds to an active and not passive process in the nervous system. This relaxation is an active process; the brain is working. So the exercises which you must do from today will not produce a state of rest, drowsiness or sleep. This is not at all what we are aiming at during your confinement, but just the opposite. We aim at maintaining, at raising, your brain's threshold of sensation; and you know very well that during sleep the threshold of sensation decreases. A person half asleep or dozing is not in a position to carry out an action. Now, you will have to direct your actions during your confinement.

What is going to be the use of this neuromuscular training and the relaxation which results from it? It is very easy to understand. During childbirth, you will have to use certain muscles in a special way and for reasons which you will be told. If you are really familiar with these muscles, and have taught them the work they have got to do, it will be easy for you to use them when the time comes. You will carry out the movements necessary in childbirth easily with greatest effect and least effort. But if you have not learnt, you will not work properly or logically; your movements will not be correct and they will not give results. This training is therefore indispensable.

It is a training in movement, purposeful movement. I have just talked about movements which are of use in childbirth. But will all your muscles be of use, all the time? Clearly not. You must also be familiar with those muscles which will not be of use at certain times in childbirth, and you must train them so that they do not work and do not interfere with the work of other muscles—notably the uterus—when there is a contraction. So, as a result of learning the useful movements and how to act to keep the muscles separate, you will achieve perfect co-ordination of motor activity. Nowadays, we should not see trained women becoming restless during contractions, because they have learnt the movements that are useful. In the past it was different. A woman once said: 'Yes, when they (the contractions) came, I shrivelled up.' She used the terms 'pains'. She was referring to contractions, but these had assumed the proportions of pain and were in fact accompanied by pain.

I am now going to explain why the pain increases and is at once followed by increasing restlessness. I advise you to make a note of the diagram which summarizes the actual principles of the training for childbirth without pain and its application.

In the third lecture, you were given an account of the nervous system, and I told you that the ratio of the forces should always be to the advantage of the brain. When the brain has a high potential, it has a good braking power, and the stimuli which come from the internal organs do not cross its threshold of sensation. To the brain we attributed a certain strength, or potential. I suggested twenty to thirty volts. Let us say that it is at twenty volts, that all the stimuli coming from the internal organs—from the vegetative nervous system—are at eight volts, and that the threshold of sensation is, therefore, not crossed.

We also saw that, after a serious emotional shock, the potential of the brain could fall, to five volts for example, while all the stimuli coming from the internal organs increased in intensity, reaching ten to twelve volts. The ration of the forces was reversed; the brain had lost its braking power. We established a relationship between all the minor shocks which affected you during pregnancy and minor shocks which may affect anyone during life, upsetting the nervous equilibrium. A severe shock might be compared with the first signs of childbirth. Suppose the continual shock which decreased the brain's braking power had been a telegram telling you that someone whom you loved had died. Suppose now that the person had been knocked down by a motor-car, and had been badly injured. She was treated but got worse. You heard of her accident; you had news of her illness. She grew worse and worse, and in the last days you knew that nothing more could be done. When you received the telegram announcing her death, would you react in the same way as in the first case? Certainly not. You were prepared for it. You knew in advance what was going to happen. At your confinement exactly the same thing will happen. You will know all about it—how it begins and goes on—and you will know also what you have to do. Thus the small shocks of pregnancy cannot affect you in the same way. You are in a position to fight, and it is in these conditions that you face childbirth—with a very high potential and your brain possessing a good braking power. Thanks to the application of everything you have learnt during training, you will maintain this nervous equilibrium throughout childbirth.

Let us return to the woman who had no training. She arrived probably for her confinement supported by her husband and her mother or mother-in-law. Then the usual last advice was given. These future mothers were afraid. They did not know how their babies would be born. And their nervous equilibrium was upset. Now the breakdown of nervous equilibrium creates a phenomenon which we have not yet mentioned—a breakdown in the equilibrium of the circulation of the blood: vasomotor disorders. Of course, all of you have turned pale or blushed; when they are young, people are very emotional and blush easily.

And when we blush, what happens? It is as though there is a small fire in your brain; the sensory threshold rises. And the heart beats more quickly; and the little vessels which pass through the skin widen. We say that vaso-dilatation occurs. The blood circulates more easily and in greater quantity; you go very red. And when we turn pale? It is exactly the opposite. When an unpleasant shock occurs, a fright for example, we go very pale because the calibre of the small vessels which pass through the skin decreases. Vasoconstriction occurs. We blush; we turn pale. What has this to do with childbirth?

What is true for the surface of our bodies is also true for the internal organs. These two phenomena—the breakdown of the nervous equilibrium followed by that of the equilibrium of the blood circulation—can have repercussions on internal organs of woman in labour. The uterus, which contains your baby, is a hollow muscle. During childbirth, as we have seen, it contracts strongly so that it does a great deal of work. A great liberation of energy results, and hence there is great combustion. But for the combustion to be complete there must be enough O_2, and the oxygen is brought to the uterus by the blood. The uterus must therefore receive enough blood to provide the quantity of O_2 necessary for the combustion. Breakdown of the equilibrium of the circulation affects the work of the uterus. This, no longer receives the amount of blood it needs and lacks oxygen. Combustion is not assured; the work cannot be done—at least not properly. Functionally, therefore, trouble will occur, because the uterus is more or less in a state of intoxication.

Thus, in childbirth without training, stimuli which leave the nerve endings in this muscle during contraction become so strong that they cross the brain's sensory threshold. They cross it especially easily as there is already a reversal of the ratio of the forces, a lowering of sensory threshold. Here then is the first effect of this sequence of events. In such conditions, contraction has assumed the character of pain; and, associated with this, the fear and dread of suffering appear. One thing leads to another. As soon as it occurs, the contraction also makes the woman restless. She clenches her fists, groans, screams, makes disordered movements and so on. There is not only motor but psycho-motor inco-ordination. Is restlessness helpful or harmful to the progress of childbirth? It is harmful. This behaviour amounts altogether to a series of useless conditioned reflexes. How can we influence all these events which form a vicious circle?

I repeat—I cannot repeat it enough—from the beginning, what you have learnt enables you to approach childbirth in the best conditions. As soon as the first signs occur, you should put this knowledge into practice. You know exactly what you should do. You respond to your contractions instead of submitting to them, and in this way you realize that they are accompanied by normal and not painful sensations. Right from the beginning your contractions will have lost the quality of pain, but they will have acquired a new quality. They will be the signal for you to begin your part—and of course what you do will depend on what you know. You must not act blindly; you must understand what you are doing. Is this activity helpful or harmful to the progress of childbirth? It is clearly helpful. It is the result of your training; of a sum of valuable conditioned reflexes.

Let us go on to a study of the exercises which you must do from today onwards. It is possible that, at the beginning, you will meet with some difficulties. This is perfectly normal when you exercise for the

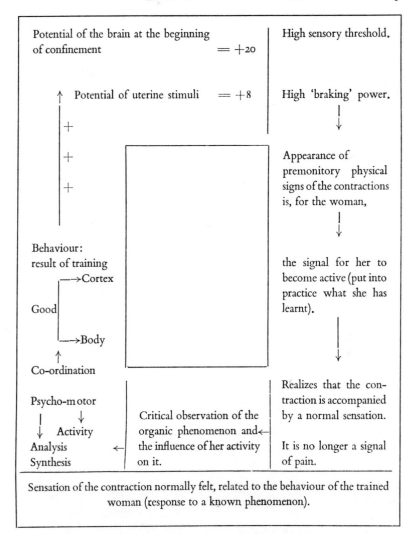

Potential of the brain at the beginning
of confinement   = +20

High sensory threshold.

↑   Potential of uterine stimuli   = +8

High 'braking' power.

+

+

+

Appearance of premonitory physical signs of the contractions is, for the woman,

Behaviour:
result of training
   —→Cortex

Good

   —→Body
↑
Co-ordination

the signal for her to become active (put into practice what she has learnt).

Psycho-motor
  | ↓
  ↓   Activity
Analysis   ←—
Synthesis

Critical observation of the organic phenomenon and←—
the influence of her activity on it.

Realizes that the contraction is accompanied by a normal sensation.

It is no longer a signal of pain.

Sensation of the contraction normally felt, related to the behaviour of the trained woman (response to a known phenomenon).

first time. When you learned to type, did you get brilliant results the first time? Certainly not. It is by repetition that you become expert. You must, therefore, repeat the exercises concerned.

Usually you will do them lying on your back ('deck chair' position, semi-recumbent); but also from time to time you will do them lying on your side, and in a sitting position. Before starting this exercise, breathe deeply. Then get the feel of your muscles one after the other, contracting them fairly strongly. This is the work of the brain showing

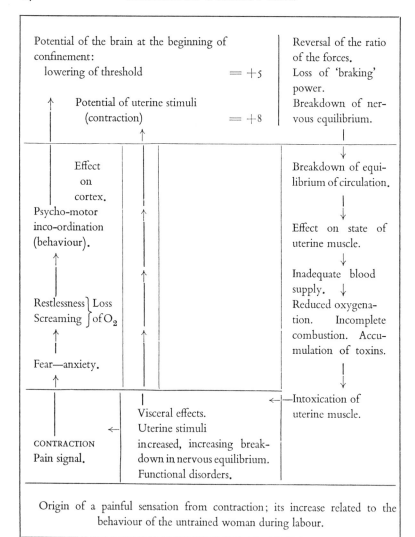

Potential of the brain at the beginning of confinement: lowering of threshold			$= +5$	Reversal of the ratio of the forces. Loss of 'braking' power.
↑ Potential of uterine stimuli (contraction) ↑			$= +8$	Breakdown of nervous equilibrium.
Effect on cortex. Psycho-motor inco-ordination (behaviour). ↑	↑	↑		↓ Breakdown of equilibrium of circulation. ↓ Effect on state of uterine muscle. ↓ Inadequate blood supply. ↓ Reduced oxygenation. Incomplete combustion. Accumulation of toxins.
Restlessness ⎱ Loss Screaming ⎰ of O₂ ↑ Fear—anxiety. ↑				↓
CONTRACTION Pain signal. ←	⎸ Visceral effects. Uterine stimuli increased, increasing breakdown in nervous equilibrium. Functional disorders.		←⎸—Intoxication of uterine muscle.	

Origin of a painful sensation from contraction; its increase related to the behaviour of the untrained woman during labour.

itself in positive motor activity. You feel your muscles one after another. You become conscious of them. Then you do exactly the opposite. You put the same muscles in a state of complete rest, relaxed, and you keep them like this throughout the exercise. Afterwards, you will control the relaxation of these different muscles one after the other. You will do this for four or five days.

After the four or five days, you begin to make the exercise more complicated. When you control one part, you must at the same time move another part. For example, if you control the relaxation of the arm or forearm, you must at the same time extend, then flex, one foot or the shoulder, hand or fingers. Repeat this for four or five days.

At the end of this time you will elaborate further, moving two parts—the feet, the forearms, the shoulders: it does not matter. Why all this? It is very easy to understand. As a result of the progressive course you follow during these various exercises, you will very quickly succeed, first in differentiating and then in separating the muscular activity that is useful from the activity that is not useful. When you reach childbirth you will be able to make the right muscles work separately and, *at the same time*, to relax the muscles which must not be used. From this progressive course of exercises you will obtain surprising results.

Let us consider delivery. Women who have followed the training can now keep certain muscles of the pelvis relaxed, expecially the muscles of the pelvic floor. These muscles take no further part, and this is the essential thing; because when they contract—and they do contract in untrained women—they obstruct the passage of the head of the baby through the vagina. This no longer happens in childbirth without pain. At the same time you are able to make other muscles work—the abdominal muscles. The way out remains free, and, as the contraction of the abdominal muscles is well controlled, delivery will be much quicker. This neuromuscular training plays an important part in childbirth. But it is only part of the training. A woman would be making a mistake if she thought that, thanks to neuromuscular training, she will obtain good relaxation and her childbirth will be painless. Several factors make up training. If you separate them they lose their value; they are no longer effective.

There are also some women who think that successful childbirth is a question of will-power. That also is wrong. You must be willing to learn and then to put the knowledge into practice. By will-power alone you could not give birth without pain. If you could, many women with a lot of will-power would have done so. Imagine that you have never learnt anything about electricity, and you knew nothing about a wireless. I put in front of you all the parts required to make a radio set and say: 'There you are. You are going to make this set by tomorrow, and it must work.' You are full of good intentions, but the next day, when I return, will the set be made? Certainly not. You do not know the technique or the principles. For childbirth, it is exactly the same thing. Knowledge, and only knowledge, enables you to act rationally. Will-power intervenes only to make you learn and apply what you have learnt. I hope that you understand the difference properly.

And now let us pass on to the exercises.

Lecture 7

Dilatation

Today I am going to talk about dilatation. You already know something about it. It answers the problem: 'How can a baby of such a size come out through such a small passage?'

Here is a diagram of the uterus seen in section. I remind you that the upper part is called the fundus. It is the fundus which comes into indirect contact with the diaphragm, bearing the pressure which this muscle exerts on the abdominal contents when it is lowered during inspiration. I have drawn the thickness of the wall which forms the fundus and the thickness of the wall of the body of the uterus. The wall ends below in a much thicker part—the cervix. The cervix closes the lower part of the uterus. It joins the uterine cavity to the vaginal cavity, and it is bounded above by what is called the internal orifice and below by the external orifice. The baby is inside the uterus, but during pregnancy his body is developing. He is continually changing, and, being very fragile, he must be protected, especially against any injury from without.

Diaphragm

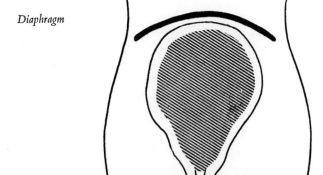

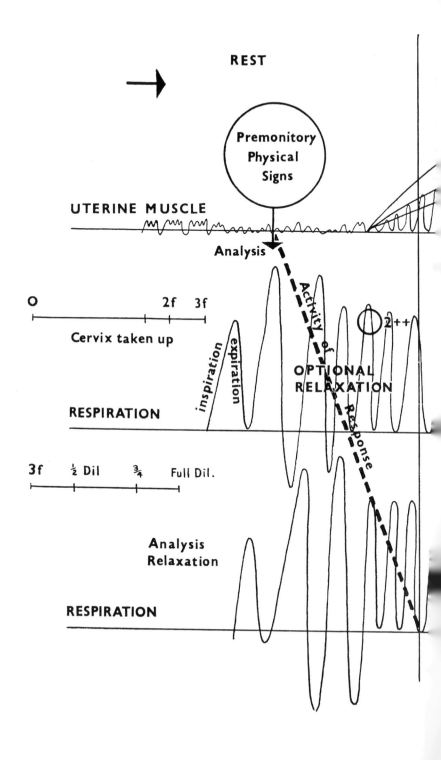

REST

Premonitory Physical Signs

UTERINE MUSCLE

Analysis

O   2f   3f

Cervix taken up

inspiration

expiration

Activity of

2++

OPTIONAL RELAXATION

Response

RESPIRATION

3f   ½ Dil   ¾   Full Dil.

Analysis Relaxation

RESPIRATION

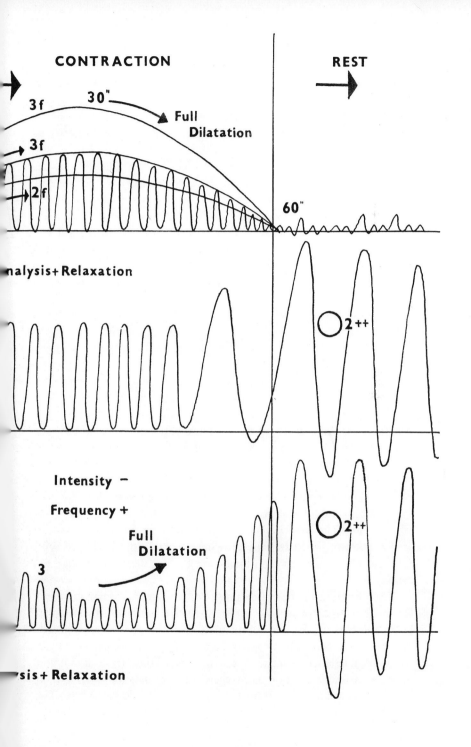

No germ or microbe must penetrate from the outside to him. The vaginal cavity remains open, and the cervix is not sufficient protection. How then is the baby protected against germs and microbes? Mainly by membranes. The cervix is some protection but only a mechanical one. It is not water-tight. These membranes, then, are in contact with the whole internal surface of the uterus, completely enclosing the baby. The baby lives in a closed bag. The membranes surround what is called the egg; we can compare them to the fine skin which is found in a new-laid egg. The membranes hold not only the baby but also the amniotic fluid. They themselves are protected at their lowest point by a gelatinous substance which collects in the passage between the internal and external orifices, thus forming the mucous plug. This term is confusing and not very appropriate. The mucous plug acts like a filter. If we examined the contents of the lowest third of it, we should discover many germs and microbes. If we examined its middle third, we should find very few, and if finally we examined the upper third, the part touching the membranes, we should find no germs at all. These, therefore, are the different ways in which the baby is protected during pregnancy.

But at childbirth these protections become obstacles which must be removed. The plug does not come out all at once like the cork out of a bottle but it disintegrates very slowly under the influence of the contractions. And when it disintegrates you lose some blood and mucus—very little blood, much less than the amount lost at your periods. The membranes also rupture, as a rule, through the effect of the contractions, letting out the amniotic fluid. You lose the waters. You can lose them all at once, or only a little at first, the rest following.

How much fluid will you lose? Between a half and two pints is a fair amount. The fluid is slightly viscous and, as a rule, it is clear. I repeat, you lose the waters any time during childbirth. I will give you more details soon. But what obstacle is left? The most important—the cervix.

The dilatation of the cervix progresses slowly. A woman in labour for the first time must expect eight to twelve hours for dilatation to become complete, for the cervix to open fully. A woman who has already had a baby can expect a considerably shorter period, six to ten hours, nearer six than ten. But do not regard these times as definite; they vary from one person to another. Also, if dilatation takes longer, it does not mean that the woman cannot give birth without pain. The length of time is significant only for the doctor or midwife. I will return to this question in a moment, because it has a considerable influence on your behaviour.

Eight to twelve hours is still quite a long time. I am going to give you the reasons. Let us try to discover the size of the cervix at term; we are going to suppose that we cut across it. We could examine it from above, and it would then appear like two small circles: a smaller one corresponding to the canal of the cervix and a bigger circle corresponding to the cervix's outer surface, with a diameter of about one and a quarter inches. The diameter of the cervix will change very greatly in relation to the diameter of the child's head, which is the biggest object to be delivered all at once. The size of the head can be regarded as irreducible. When dilatation is complete, the two diameters are equal, that of the cervix and that of the head. But this means that the entire cervical tissue gradually expands to reach full

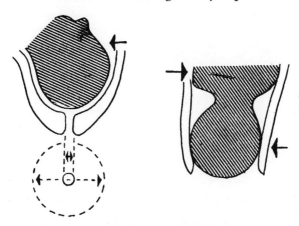

dilatation. Dilatation means the stretching of all the tissues which form the cervix, and for this to take place normally and physiologically a certain time is necessary. Time is needed for organic changes to occur, acting on the tissues, allowing them to stretch. There are roughly two kinds of organic changes.

1. *Chemical changes*, resulting from the intermittent production of hormones—chemical substances which are taken up by the tissues and which modify them. They soften the tissues and allow them to respond to the second type of changes.

2. *Mechanical changes*. Though dilatation of the cervix is slow and progressive, it is not continuous, but *interrupted*. The cervix opens only during the contractions. This is the aim of the contractions, which act

mechanically on the cervical tissues but only after these have been softened by the hormones. When the contraction is finished, the cervix tends to return nearly to its previous position, which means that it loses much of the ground gained. I emphasize the interrupted nature of the process. Your work is confined to the contractions. So that, although ten to fifteen hours are necessary for the cervix to open, the real work amounts to two to three hours only. This completely changes your views of childbirth. Having carried your baby and thought about his birth for nine months, you will have two or three

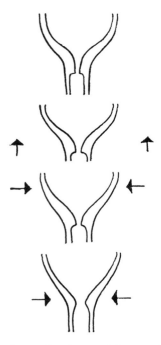

hours of serious work to do during labour—the response to your contractions.

How do these contractions work? The uterus is roughly formed of two kinds of muscle fibres. Some are vertically placed, directed towards the top, and distributed, of course, throughout the wall of the uterus. Others go around the uterus and are called the circular muscle fibres. So, there are longitudinal and circular fibres, which contract at the same time. Each time the longitudinal fibres contract, they pull the cervix upwards. At each contraction, the cervix gradually rises towards the uterus, thanks to the suppleness it has just acquired. The cervix, at the beginning, becomes thinner and is taken up to become part of the uterus, and is incorporated in the lower segment. It is so well incorporated that, once dilatation is complete, the cervix and the body of the uterus blend into each other and are indistinguishable.

The muscle fibres contract at the same time as the longitudinal fibres, but they merely act as a support. They cannot be regarded as working dynamically; they maintain the shape of the uterus. The longitudinal fibres work at the same time, and so the fundus of the uterus is lowered. The uterus decreases in height. Great pressure is then applied to its contents—the baby, the fluid and the placenta. The volume of the fluid does not change during pressure; but the bag which holds the fluid can stretch. The membranes will give way at a certain place—in the lower part. At each contraction, the membranes will be pushed into the vaginal cavity, which is an advantage. So much for the fluid.

Let us now turn to the baby. Pressure is going to be exerted on him too. You know that the baby's head is usually here, in the lower part. As the fundus of the uterus is lowered and its height decreases, the baby is pushed towards the way out, and quite a strong pressure will be exerted through the head on the internal orifice of the cervix.

Clearly, if we compare the direction of the two arrows, we see that one force is exerted vertically upwards, and the other vertically downwards. You would think these two forces would neutralize each other. But they add to each other. They are not exerted at the same place in the uterus. One is outside; the other inside. If the baby presents as a breech the result will be the same. If you like, it is a little less pleasant to push with the breech than with the head.

These different changes are accompanied by physical sensations. You should know about them so that you can understand the use of the contraction, how it appears and progresses. You must observe these physical sensations carefully. How is the work of the longitudinal fibres felt? As a pull, having the pubis as a starting point, or in any case near the pubis, perhaps a little above or a little below. A very distinct pull is exerted in this region. Perhaps you have already noticed it if you have tried to analyse the contractions carefully, as we asked you to in the third lecture. Immediately afterwards, this pulling sensation will diffuse to the right and left towards the groins. Then it reaches the front of the uterus, while the contraction increases in intensity.

The work of the circular fibres shows itself as a pressure that the woman feels during the contractions after labour has been going on for a certain time. You will be asked—by the doctor and midwife—what direction the pressure of the head is taking. You should give as precise an answer as possible, because, from what you tell us and also from our own observations, we may ask you to change your position. Do not confuse the pressure of your baby's head with the feeling of heaviness that you may feel towards the end of pregnancy. This feeling is continuous, while the pressure of the head occurs only during contraction, and as a rule after labour has been going on for a certain time.

I have told you how the contractions act and emphasized that the cervix becomes thinner and is taken up. After that, it will open and increase in diameter, which is measured in finger-widths. You will not be surprised if, after the first examination, you are told that you are two fingers dilated. That will simply mean that the cervix is open to the width of two fingers.

The stages of dilatation are one, two and three fingers. Three fingers is still not enough to allow the head to pass through, and dilatation will continue. After three fingers, we say the cervix becomes half dilated, then three-quarters dilated, and finally, fully dilated.

You must remember these terms, since we divide dilatation into two parts. The first part extends from no dilatation to three fingers, and the second, from then until full dilatation, passing through half and three-quarters dilatation. The first phase is much the slower. If twelve hours were necessary, for example, for the whole dilatation, reckon on eight or nine hours for the first phase. Of these eight or nine hours, five or six are needed for the cervix to be taken up. You may arrive at the maternity home when dilatation has just begun and, when you are examined again three or four hours later, the cervix may still be being taken up. Do not conclude, 'At this rate, I shan't have my baby until January and it's only September.' The second phase is much quicker.

How long do contractions last during labour? Between twenty seconds and one minute. For some women, the contractions do not last as long at the beginning of labour as at the end. For an equal number, the contractions last the same time throughout. Whether or not you remember what I have just told you is of minor importance because we are going to assume that all the contractions last one minute. During your labour, you will have to react *at the moment* of the contractions. You will have to do some exercises which, when the time comes, will enable you to respond to your contractions. This is why we choose, from now on, the longer rather than the shorter duration. A contraction does not reach its peak straight away; it starts unobtrusively. Then, little by little, it increases in intensity, reaches its highest point, stays there a few seconds, then begins to diminish, and disappears. During the first thirty seconds the contraction becomes stronger and during the last thirty seconds it becomes weaker.

The interval between contractions varies greatly. Some women at the beginning of their labour may have thirty-minute intervals and others six- or seven-minute intervals. The duration of labour, however, does not depend on the length of interval. In the first three hours the contractions become steady, and the intervals between them become equal. Their strength increases as labour progresses. At half dilatation, the contractions reach maximum strength. They increase no more, but, at full dilatation, they change their quality. At half dilatation the interval between them is shortest—as a rule three minutes.

I am now going to show you the curve of the tone of the uterine muscle during and between contractions. A few words, first of all, on what we call muscular tone. A muscle changes in consistency according to whether it works or rests. A muscle at rest is soft and supple. We say that its tone is weak. When a muscle works it has a firm consistency. Our muscles are full of vibrations. When they are at rest, these are weak and infrequent. During activity, they are strong and frequent.

These vibrations of our muscles can be recorded with rather complicated technical apparatus, but this is not important for us because the principle of recording is very simple. Every time a vibration occurs in the muscle, the pen jumps on the paper. We call this an oscillation, and the larger the vibration the larger is the oscillation. The tracing of all these waves gives a general curve which I am going to show on the diagram.

These vibrations can very easily be heard. There is no need for any apparatus, and you have certainly heard the vibration of some of your muscles. In bed, if it is very quiet and your head is buried in the pillow, you must have heard a crackling in your ear when you clenched your teeth. These are the jaw muscles that you hear because you have just contracted them very strongly. In case you have not noticed this, do it tonight when you go to bed. Put your head on the pillow and clench your teeth.

But let us return to our diagram. The time is in this direction. Here we are during rest—small vibrations. A very small movement of the needle. Another vibration, still another very small one—you see, the intensity is really very weak. Now we reach the contractions. At once these vibrations increase in intensity. Remember what we have just said: first thirty seconds curve rising; second thirty seconds curve falling. And the vibrations multiply and increase in intensity. They are now frequent. It is the peak of the contraction. Then they decrease in intensity, and we go back to the previous curve—weak vibrations, weak oscillations, and so on. We have chosen a time in the middle of labour, with between two and three fingers of dilatation. If I had wanted to show the tone and vibrations of the muscle during the preceding period, we should have a lower curve. This is what it would look like. If, on the other hand, I had wanted to show the intensity of contractions between three fingers and full dilatation, we should have a higher curve. All this is very simple.

Your behaviour should differ according to the phases of labour. You will not have to do the same things at the beginning as after three-fingers dilatation or as at the end of dilatation. To know what you will do during the period of rest, we are going to find out what women used to do between contractions, when they had no training. They were thinking of the next contraction—of a pain, the next pain. They dreaded it. The contraction had assumed the quality of a pain, and they were afraid. Their nervous system continued to suffer between contractions and the shocks to it increased. The sensory threshold of their brain continued to fall, and the ratio of the forces to be reversed. There was no real period of rest between contractions for these women.

For you the same problems no longer arise. Your knowledge will enable you to approach confinement with your nervous system in a good state of equilibrium. From the beginning of labour, by putting into practice all you have been taught, you will realize that the contractions are not accompanied by pain, that this sensation is not painful. You will not be dreading the next pain, since there will not have been one before. You will have to think of the next contraction, but not passively. You will try two objectives:

1. To respond better and better to the contractions. If everything goes perfectly, there is no problem, but if there is a small hitch—this can happen—you must try to understand why, and ask the people in attendance to help.

2. To avoid wasting your energy. You must try, from a certain stage of labour (about three fingers), to recover the maximum energy in the minimum time.

During a contraction, you will have to keep working both mentally and physically. You should participate consciously in it. The more you know about it, the better you will follow its progress, and the better will you respond and adapt. By this only will you get results. You must notice carefully how the contraction appears, develops and disappears, at least after a certain stage has been reached.

During labour, as in the training, you must never work mechanically or automatically. We do a thing well only if we know why we do it. During a contraction you will test the efficiency of your training. Physically, your work will consist of breathing quickly and shallowly, and of keeping your abdominal and pelvic-floor muscles completely relaxed. We shall consider this relaxation in the next lecture.

We ask you to breathe like this and to maintain this relaxation to give the uterus the best possible conditions to work in. This muscle, in fact, feels every bit of pressure, as do all the hollow organs. The shallow quick breathing is intended to limit the extent of the movements of the diaphragm. The breathing is superficial and at the same time rapid in order to maintain good oxygenation. And, finally, the abdominal and pelvic-floor muscles must be relaxed so that the lateral walls and the lower part of the uterus (the cervix and the lower segment) are not subjected to any pressure. The fundus is thus free, and so are the sides and the lower segment.

It is upon this shallow rapid breathing that we put special emphasis. As a rule, it is only helpful from three fingers dilatation. Before this, you must breathe from time to time, between contractions. Then breathe out more deeply, say twice in succession. Then resume normal breathing and keep it up throughout the contraction, and so on. As soon as the contraction has stopped, you must breathe in and blow out deeply several times in succession to take in plenty of oxygen. The number of times depends entirely on how much you need.

From three fingers dilatation—it may be a little before or a little after—the rule is the same as in the previous period. Between contractions, from time to time breathe deeply so as to keep well oxygenated: then return to normal breathing. When the contraction arrives, breathe much less deeply and, at the same time, greatly speed up the breathing.

The curve corresponds to the one shown for the contraction, but it is the opposite on the diagram—less strong but quicker, and at the peak of the contraction your breathing will be really shallow and rapid. Then the contraction diminishes and the breathing returns to normal. When the contraction is finished use deep inspiration, deep expiration, several times in succession.

There are three important points to remember.

1. This breathing, which is accompanied by relaxation, should start a few seconds before the contraction. There are what are called 'premonitory' physical signs of the contractions, and you must try to detect them in the first part of labour, when the contractions are not strong and labour is easy. The most frequent sign is a movement occurring in any part of the uterus. The contraction occurs a few moments after this wave has stopped. The contraction is sometimes preceded by a movement of the baby. This happens less often, but it is more obvious.

There is still another sign—a very transient acceleration of the heart. In trained women, we do not now notice this acceleration. In untrained women a certain amount of fatigue has to be compensated for and the heart beats more quickly. You can also manage to start at the right moment if you have an idea of the interval between contractions. Not all women succeed in detecting these premonitory signs; and this can cause serious difficulties. The contraction will first take you by surprise and will be accompanied by an unpleasant sensation; then, when it next happens, it will be accompanied by a sensation of difficulty and finally of pain. It will again have assumed the quality of a pain signal.

In case of difficulty, you must ask the assistants to help you. You must be observant, discuss and exchange ideas with them. Their experience is there to assist you. Then everything will come back to normal. Thanks to this team-work, you can soon detect one of these premonitory signs and integrate your response with them.

2. If the membranes break at the beginning, it does not have much effect on the rhythm or strength of the contractions. Women say, 'I have lost the waters.' But usually they break at about three fingers dilatation. And, if not, they are ruptured artificially in most cases; the doctor or midwife does this during a contraction since the membranes are pushed into the vaginal cavity and are then easy to reach. This procedure is quite painless. As soon as the membranes rupture, the

fluid comes out. Usually the head then presses on the internal orifice of the cervix, and you feel the pressure we have just talked about. The contractions become stronger and closer together, which means that you have to go through a more critical period of adaptation. If you are not sure that you can respond, you must at once tell the assistant and make her help you. Do not let yourself be overwhelmed by what is happening.

3. The third important point concerns the period which precedes full dilatation. The quality of your contractions changes once more and your behaviour must change also. A completely different phase now begins. The purpose of the contractions until then was to open the cervix. Now this is almost done, and the contractions now aim at starting the delivery of the baby. The muscular fibres around the cornua, as well as the circular fibres, come into action and help delivery.

For the first time you will feel a desire to push. It is an absolute reflex, starting in the uterus to help its work. At first you feel it very little. It becomes more obvious at each contraction, and is very strong when you are fully dilated. But you may suddenly want to push at the beginning of delivery. As soon as you feel this desire to push, whether it appears gradually or suddenly, you must tell the assistant, and you must not push. How do you avoid it? This will be explained to you in the next lecture.

Relaxation is required throughout in the periods of rest except from the beginning until three-fingers dilatation. In this period, you need not maintain complete relaxation, but you can if you like. On the other hand it is essential at a contraction, especially for the abdominal and pelvic-floor muscles. We shall deal with all this next time. From three-fingers dilatation, the relaxation is required between contractions because of the rule: 'Recover the maximum strength in the minimum time'; and of course it is also required during contractions. Maintain good relaxation of the abdominal and pelvic-floor muscles but you must also keep the muscles of the neck and shoulders completely relaxed—as well as the back and the buttocks. I have not talked about the arms or the legs, but that does not mean that you should move them about. If the neck and shoulder muscles are well relaxed, the arms follow suit; and if the back and buttock muscles are also well relaxed, the legs are too. You will have no difficulty at all.

The exercise which you now have to do consists of shallow, rapid breathing, accompanied by complete relaxation. It is an application of the principle taught during the lecture on neuromuscular training. Cerebral activity is converted into positive motor activity—breathing, and into 'negative' activity—relaxation. To obtain a perfect result, perfect psycho-motor activity, you must train yourself seriously. If you think that you can achieve this result without preparation and training you are mistaken.

You should do this exercise lying down, usually on your back. Also do it sitting down, and lying on your side. At first, do not overdo it, and do not try to do it too long. Remember that the contractions last only twenty to thirty seconds. Repeat this exercise in the following two days—six times during the day and twenty or thirty seconds each time. After three days, still do it six times, but for twenty-five or thirty-five seconds each time and so on. When you can keep it up for one minute, carry on four times daily until confinement.

I advise you also to breathe not too superficially nor too rapidly at the beginning. Further, the breathing must be begun when your lungs are neither too full nor too empty. The best moment is at the end of the passive phase of expiration. Remember the exercise which you learned at the end of the second lecture. You had to breathe deeply, then open the mouth to let the air out passively, and, when the pressures were equal, blow at the candle. Today, instead of blowing at the candle, you must begin to breathe in a little less deeply and expel the air completely. Always return to the end of the passive phase, which corresponds exactly to the curve which I have just drawn for you on the blackboard. If you breathe like this, you will have no difficulty. You will not come back next time and say: 'I felt I was suffocating or bursting' or 'I felt dizzy.' You can breathe either through the nose or the mouth. It may be a bit more difficult through the nose, because the nasal passages are not so free, but it has the advantage of not making you thirsty as breathing through the mouth does. In any case, you will have something to drink during labour. You will be asked to rinse your mouth, then drink—a mouthful of ordinary water or mineral water, with a bit of lemon that you can bring. They will also give you tea, which is a very good stimulant for the nervous system. And this procedure, rinsing the mouth and taking a mouthful of liquid, is repeated as often as you like, thus avoiding the evil effects of that antiquated custom of forbidding you to drink. It resulted in loss of energy through dehydration. A thirsty person thinks only of one thing—that she is thirsty; and, when she has drunk, she thinks that she was thirsty, in any case, she was dehydrated and unable to make an effort. You will also be made comfortable. In the past, this aspect was completely neglected and it was thought that the woman should lie on something hard, a wooden or metal table—of course not directly on the wood or metal, but all the same it was very hard. If you asked why, they would have said because you must.

Lecture 8

Delivery

D ELIVERY is the period of labour which you will find the most interesting.

You will consciously follow its progress, knowing at each moment what you must do. It is the time when you will have to produce your greatest efforts. They do not last long, but are quite intense. This period, which nowadays leaves you with the most moving memories, was, in the past, the most dreaded of the whole confinement. Women without real knowledge, and sometimes completely ignorant, could not see how to resolve satisfactorily the terrible problem of delivery. The size of the baby is out of all proportion to the size of the possible ways out. Most women, in talking of confinement, were thinking of the period of delivery only. But to make delivery physiologically and mechanically possible the disproportion which we have just noted must be corrected.

This is what happens during dilatation of the cervix of the uterus, the first stage of labour. For you, it is no longer a mystery. When dilatation is ended the contractions change in quality, and you feel an absolute reflex arising in the uterus. You feel a desire to push.

Delivery is beginning. You will use the strength available to you to overcome the final resistance. You will voluntarily help your uterus to expel the infant which it contains.

In the past, when women felt this desire to push, it was a moment of panic for them because they did not know how to push. They had to be taught, and the doctors and midwives then resorted to a makeshift arrangement. Those of you who have already had a baby will remember what you were told. At the moment when they were going to deliver their baby, they received this astonishing order: 'Push. Like opening your bowels.' Such an order could not correspond with the needs of that moment. When you push in opening your bowels, you use the muscles which together form what is called the pelvic floor.

The pelvis is made up of two bones—the iliac bones. They are large blades, which, as they turn, slope down and join together in front and below at the pubis. They are joined at the back through another bone, formed of five vertebrae very firmly fixed to each other—the sacrum: the whole makes up the pelvis, a sort of basin sloping downwards and forwards. The pelvis is pierced in its central lower part, and this free space is called the pelvic outlet. It is through this outlet that the baby must pass before it is delivered. Now it is closed, obstructed, by the muscles of the pelvic floor.

Thus, we have a bony surround, and the bottom of the basin is obstructed. But this does not make up the lower limit of the body. Beneath the pelvic floor there are still other organs, nerves and vessels, and passages pass through. These nerves and vessels do not interest us much, but the passages do. There are two. At the back, the rectum, which passes at first along the vertebral column, continues in the rectal ampulla and ends at the anal orifice. In front of the rectum is the second passage—the vaginal cavity, which ends at the vulva. Rectum at the back; vagina in the front. When you push to open the bowels, the muscles of the pelvic floor contract slowly. At the back, they compress the rectum, which is perfect for meeting the completely normal and physiological needs of defaecation. But in a woman, as these muscles compress the rectum behind, so they compress the vagina just as strongly!

Thus a woman who pushes in this way during labour creates an obstacle to the passage of her baby through the vagina. This effort not only fails to meet the needs of the moment, but is contrary to them. You must not push like this. Of course, the baby is born nevertheless. He manages to cross this obstacle, simply because the three forces together—the contraction of the uterus, the work of the abdominal muscles and the pressure of the diaphragm—make up a force greater than the constriction of the vaginal cavity by the muscles of the pelvic floor. But the obstacle is crossed by force, which means that the woman has to produce much stronger and especially much more prolonged efforts.

Now we know that delivery must of necessity be quick. Furthermore, in nearly all cases, a hardening, a reflex tension, develops in the perineum, and this itself presents difficulties. It is very unfortunate because, during delivery, the head of the baby leaves the uterus, presses behind on the tissues of the perineum, and, as it progresses, pushes all the tissues in front of itself. These tissues gradually become quite considerably stretched; but only under one condition. For a tissue to become stretched, it must remain elastic. Now where women push wrongly these tissues lose their elasticity and create an obstacle to the good progress of the head. You can understand why women are torn. These muscles and tissues cannot stretch, and a moment arrives when they give way.

I repeat. You must not push as in opening the bowels. You must realize that it is a matter of driving a baby out and nothing else. If, from now on, you try to keep a clear idea of the position of the baby in your uterus, of the position of the uterus in your abdomen, then you will understand where the expulsive forces must be exerted. You will understand at the same time where they should not be exerted. You must know beforehand what the act of delivering a baby consists of. It would be nonsense to exert the expulsive forces, as they used to be exerted, in the region of the vagina and the rectum. The passage must remain free. The expulsive forces are exerted slightly on the sides and especially from the fundus towards the way out.

When must you push? When the contractions begin to be accompanied by the desire and only after you have been examined and told to push. As a rule, you should push only at the moment when the contraction reaches its maximum and not during the whole contraction. Usually your efforts last, in all, between 15 and 25 seconds, and you are asked, as a rule, to make two for each contraction. If, for example, the contraction lasts 25 seconds at its peak, you should push twice in succession: 10 or 12 seconds for the first, 10 or 12 seconds for the second.

As soon as the contraction stops, the desire to push also stops. You must not push any more. At this stage in labour, a period of one to four minutes elapses, and you must take advantage of it.

You will help the uterus by using the muscles which you know about: the diaphragm and the abdominal muscles. The diaphragm falls in inspiration and presses on the fundus of the uterus, and this pressure is directed vertically from above downwards. When delivery begins, the pressure exerted by the diaphragm on the fundus becomes very helpful. It was not so during dilatation, for the excellent reason that the way out was not free and that you did not want to push. As soon as the way out is free, you feel the desire to push; and from that moment, pressure on the fundus acts in the same direction as the uterine contraction itself, thus helping the uterus do its work.

There is no contradiction of what you were taught in the last lecture about the shallow rapid respiration. The rule is as follows: before making an effort to lower the diaphragm, you must breathe in well but not very deeply. Then you must hold your breath to hold the diaphragm down, and immobilize it in this position, so that it presses on the uterus. But this is only a part of the action. The main thing is that the diaphragm, immobilized in this low position, keeps the ribs fixed for the abdominal muscles to pull on. They can then strongly compress the abdominal contents.

I explained that the diaphragm, as it falls, throws the thoracic cage forward. The thoracic cage is big, and when it is fixed the abdominal muscles have a good point to work from efficiently. What I have just described is a common everyday matter. When one wishes to make a big effort, if, for example, I asked you to lift that table which is very heavy, what would you do? You would hold your breath. During labour, the principle is the same. And if I were now to ask you, after you have breathed in and held your breath to make your abdominal muscles work to drive out the baby, could you do it? Obviously not. At this moment, you have no desire to push. Also labour is not a daily occurrence, and the muscles are not trained for such work. We must train them, so that when the time of delivery comes you will produce very effective efforts without difficulty.

I am going to give you a description of the effort you will have to produce, and you will think that this is impossible. Do not worry. In practice, it is much easier. With our technique all women can produce the effort properly. So do not worry while you listen to the theory. After breathing in, then blowing out, then breathing in and holding it, you will be asked to make your abdominal muscles move at their upper end—the part situated near the ribs. This movement compresses the fundus of the uterus, and you will have to direct this pressure vertically from above downwards, and gently from the front to the back, so that the resultant force is directed towards the way out. This seems impossible, as I said. But you will realize how easy it is in practice. Before asking you to repeat this exercise at home, I am going to ask you to make two other completely different efforts; you will also repeat them at home throughout pregnancy, though they will not be of any use during labour.

First, having breathed in, blown out, breathed in and held it, push exactly as you would to open your bowels. Second, after you have breathed in, blown out, breathed in and held it, push exactly as you would to pass urine. You have not come here to learn these efforts but to try to understand what happens.

As regards the pelvic floor, when you make the effort to defaecate, you feel a movement occurring behind and below—that is in all the parts which surround the rectum. When you push to pass water (micturition), you feel a movement, still in the pelvic floor, this time in front and below, in all the parts which surround the bladder.

During these two efforts, the abdominal muscles work without producing any movement. We say that they work statically. They have no dynamic rôle but they serve to keep the abdominal contents in place. But in labour you must move the abdominal muscles. The first point of these defaecation and micturition exercises, which are of no use in labour, is that you will be able to notice a difference in the work of the abdominal muscles in these different efforts. Each time you analyse them, you will understand how the abdominal muscles work and why these two efforts are to be avoided. And when you produce the useful effort, on the other hand, you will be conscious of the muscles, and will use the abdominal muscles properly.

And each time you produce the two efforts, you will be conscious of the muscles of the pelvic floor. These are the muscles which we use very often during the day. At the end of your pregnancy you will know exactly what to do to keep the muscles which must not act completely relaxed. They will not interfere, and the way out will stay free during contraction. The abdominal muscles will be able to help the uterus efficiently, and delivery will be much quicker.

We will try to see how things appear in the labour ward. In the period before delivery, you are under observation, you are examined. We know very well if delivery is near or not. Then we revise with you all the movements which you must carry out. If in spite of these instructions you make a mistake during the first and second contractions, we will tell you and show you what you did wrong. You yourself will be aware of it, because you have been trained. You will be told: 'Correct it in such and such a way,' so that after the third or fourth contraction, at the most, everything will be in order and your efforts will begin to work. But this depends on your breathing reflexes—and the efficacy of your pushing depends much more on direction than on power, contrary to what was believed in the past.

Let us now discuss the breathing reflexes. Before pushing, you must breathe in, blow out deeply and fairly quickly the first time; then again breathe in not too much, and hold the breath, closing the mouth, but keeping your eyes open. You must be very attentive; be aware all the time of what we do and notice the instructions which the assistants may give by signs. Each time you push, you will realize that, thanks to your efforts, your baby is making progress towards life, that his head comes down more and more easily. In the past the term 'to give birth' was meaningless. You did not give birth; you submitted to labour and delivery. Today you will truly give birth. You will realize that it is because of you that your baby comes into the world. When you feel the effect of your effort, you will be encouraged to produce a still better one at the next contraction. You will fully and consciously experience all this, and your baby will not be placed in your arms after somebody else has brought him into the world.

When the contraction stops, the desire to push stops too and you must not push any more. One to four minutes elapse between contractions. What must be done during this time? You must keep in mind the rule 'Recover the maximum strength in the minimum time.' The first thing to do is to supply yourself with oxygen. Do not forget that you are making very great efforts without breathing, though they may not last long.[1] So that at the end of an effort, you are very flushed and congested, and you may even be a bit cyanosed, which means that you are a little asphyxiated. All the reserves of oxygen have been used up, and you need to obtain it very quickly. As soon as the contraction and your effort are finished, you must breathe in and blow out several times in succession and very deeply. I strongly advise you to concentrate on expiration, which means getting rid of as much carbon dioxide as possible. In this phase of labour, you receive oxygen artificially. At inspiration, the oxygen mask is placed on your face. It is a very small plastic mask. It is removed in expiration; then put on again in inspiration and so on. You rapidly obtain oxygen; it is not difficult. But in order to recover properly, you should remember another rule—*relaxation*. When the effort is ended, you must not remain in the position of effort. After a big effort one tends to remain tense in this position; and this was particularly true for women in labour in the past. So, complete relaxation. The shoulders and the head fall back on the pillow. The back rests on the bed. The legs are fully relaxed. Do not forget the arms. On each side of the bed you have stirrup bars to hold. When your effort is finished you should let them go, the arms then resting on the bed.

[1] We are thinking of modifying the actual technique of the effort. We believe that if training were started early enough, women could produce very effective efforts while continuing to breathe.

For quick recovery of maximum strength use oxygen and relaxation. Prepare yourself for the next contraction. But suppose that something has not gone very well. Tell the assistant about it. You should remain in close touch with her to the end. You can always discuss anything. Do not forget that we make a team.[1]

Another contraction is coming. The desire to push returns. Soon the baby's head will be seen, and you will be told when it appears at the vulva. When the head is seen, you will be told that your baby has brown hair. Do not worry. It is always brown at this stage. Then you hear the words: 'I can see your baby's head,' and you feel like producing a still greater effort. Again you push. Again it makes progress, and still more of the head is seen. The contraction stops and you recover. Another contraction, another effort, and the head advances. Soon, during another contraction, the head will be ready to come out. You will feel that as a result of a very small effort on your part you can free your baby's head. The desire to push is very strong.

At this very moment you will hear the astonishing order: 'Stop pushing.' When in the past women were told this, they wondered what was happening. They thought immediately that something abnormal had occurred. The desire to push was so strong and the woman felt so clearly that she could free the baby's head that she panicked and usually went on pushing. But today you know exactly why you are given this order, and also how to carry it out. How not to push is very simple. It was and is today a matter of having a respiratory reflex which prevents you from pushing.

You know this reflex. When you push, the abdominal muscles must have something to pull on—the ribs immobilized by holding the breath. So, when you are not to push, the ribs must move so that the abdominal muscles have nothing to pull on. You have to breathe for the time it takes for the head to be delivered—about one to three minutes. The sort of breathing you have to use is between normal respiration and the shallow rapid breathing. You breathe like this for one to three minutes, sometimes less, sometimes more, and, during this time, the head is delivered.

I will explain why you must not push. During delivery, the head of the baby descends through the pelvis, and, as it descends, it turns. At each contraction, the head progresses. Now, when this contraction has stopped, the head does not stay still. It goes back up slightly;

[1] Be careful not to have a rigid system. The woman knows best in what position her effort is most effective.

so that all the tissues of the perineum, which are involved during contraction when the head progresses, relax after the contraction. The principle is the same during dilatation. Then, when contraction occurs, the cervix opens, and, when it stops, the cervix tends to return to its previous position. During delivery, the perineal tissues do the same. Of course some ground is always gained. Let us say that there is one to two inches progress and that, after the contraction, the head goes back up, but only loses about an inch.

But each time the head moves on, it turns; and at a given moment it will be completely turned around in relation to your body. The baby's face will be turned towards the vertebral column, and the nape of the neck towards your abdomen. The head moves on as a result of progress made inch by inch, and then the back of the head stops behind the pubis. The back of the head is thus stopped, and it cannot go on or back. But the face is not held up, and continues to move along the posterior wall of the vagina which is concave. The back of the head is held up on the pubis, which acts as a point of rotation and the head straightens out, or, as we say, is unflexed. But as soon as it is stopped behind the pubis, it cannot go back between contractions.

The tissues of the perineum are then well stretched. There is still a little way to go. This distance must be crossed slowly. One to three minutes are sufficient for the biggest diameter of the head to come out, to pass through the perineum. This will be achieved while you breathe, which stops you from pushing. If you push all at once, you risk being torn even if the tissues do remain fully elastic. This part of delivery must not be forced. It must not damage you.

Today we almost never touch the baby's head. We no longer direct its delivery as in the past. No doubt there are still cases where one is obliged to intervene, but if possible we avoid touching the tissues of the perineum. You will feel the delivery of your baby's head. You will be told what is happening and feel how the head presents and is delivered. We will tell you when the hair appears. You will feel the forehead slide at the back along your perineum; then the eyes, nose, mouth, and chin. When this is out, the perineum falls back, and we regard the battle as won, because the head is the largest thing there is to deliver all at once, and it is irreducible in size. But the delivery is not finished. The body and the legs remain. Naturally the shoulders are bigger than the head, but they are mobile. Their size is easily reduced; and they can be delivered one after the other.

When the head is delivered, we intervene. It is turned a good quarter of a circle, either from right to left or from left to right, depending on the presentation of the baby. This rotation of the head is followed by a rotation of the body. The aim is to bring the front shoulder under the pubis. The shoulder is there. We pull the head gently to and fro several times. In this way, progress is made. More and more of the shoulder appears until the arm-pit can be reached and at the same time gently pulled. The shoulder then comes out. We go on gently pulling the head, and the arm gradually appears. We take hold of the elbow and bring out the forearm, and then the hand.

When the hand is delivered, the arm which is free extends, usually quite strongly, so that you will feel your baby touch you for the first time. We then proceed to free the other shoulder. We hold the baby's head and raise it. Now you can see your infant for the first time. As the head is raised, you see the child in front of you, although it is still not completely delivered, and you will feel the delivery of the posterior shoulder occurring very gently. The part of the body next to it, then the arm, the forearm, the rest of the body, the hand, and finally the pelvis and the legs will follow without any difficulty. Your baby will then be given to you still joined to you by the cord. We give him to you, without saying anything, so that you will be the first to see if you have a boy or girl. This, too, is part of the training. We think that you should be the first to know the result of your efforts. To benefit from this moment, which you will never forget, you should be fully conscious, and have fully participated in labour.

The method you are taught here aims at making you conscious of what you are doing and also at improving the relationships between you and us, between women and the medical profession. In the past, it was not very interesting in human terms to observe a confinement, whereas today it is interesting. You should not think that the emotions which you experience are not shared. They are, and we never get used to them. There are as many different cases as there are women. We experience your labour with you, and this improvement in our relationship is an excellent thing.

When the baby is born, he is placed on your stomach on which a sterile cloth has been spread. You must not touch him. You may then experience two emotions—fear, very quickly followed by pleasure. You will perhaps see your baby become purple—cyanosed. This is quite normal and usually, when the child is placed on your stomach, he has not yet breathed. The blood which brought him oxygen comes to him through the cord. In the cord, if you touch it, you clearly feel the pulsations getting weaker and soon stopping completely. The blood does not reach him any more. He is immediately in a state of asphyxia. This asphyxia is physiological, we say. At that moment, the baby's blood becomes full of CO_2, and this excess of carbon dioxide stimulates bulbar centres for the first time. The stimulation is transmitted to the diaphragm through the phrenic nerve. And then you will have a pleasant experience. You will see your baby's chest begin to flutter. It will quiver, then all at once you will see it swell. The baby breathes in for the first time, and as it blows the air out it gives its first cry. A few moments later, the cord is tied in two places and cut. From then on, the life of your baby no longer depends directly on you. His independent life, his life as an infant human being, begins.

And now we will go on to the exercises. From today you have two series to do. The first consists of making efforts like opening the bowels and passing urine, exercises to be done lying down. You should do these two exercises thinking clearly about the reasons why you do them. Observe in particular the work of the muscles of the pelvic floor, and of the abdominal muscles. You make these efforts so that you can avoid them during labour. You will repeat them twice a day, and, each time, you will do them twice. Do not overdo them, of course.

This is how you should proceed for the other exercise, which will be used in labour. Lie down, and with two fingers only feel your abdomen in the pit of the stomach—the region right in the middle below the ribs and over the fundus of the uterus. You will notice that this area remains relatively soft. After having located it, still lying down, you bring your chin on to your chest without forcing it. Make this forward flexion of the head and of the cervical spine; and you will notice that this region, which was relatively soft, becomes very hard. The technique I previously mentioned, which enables you to push properly, consists precisely in bringing and keeping the chin on the chest: but this is not the only technique and we will return to this shortly. To bring the chin on to the chest while lying down you must possess abdominal muscles; if an individual had no abdominal muscles or they were paralysed, she could not do this. When you make this movement, the abdominal muscles immediately contract. Their aim is to fix the thoracic cage, to the upper part of which most of the muscles which flex the head and cervical spine are attached. If the thoracic cage is not fixed, the flexion is impossible. When the pregnant woman makes this movement lying down, the upper part of her abdominal muscles contract, pressing on the fundus of the uterus. The pressure is directed vertically from above downwards and also slightly from the front to the back. This corresponds exactly to what is needed, and there is no woman incapable of carrying out this movement. All women can push more or less properly, sometimes perhaps not very well, but never badly.

Before an expulsive effort you must breathe in, blow out deeply and quite quickly, breathe in, not too much, stop by closing the mouth, and keep your eyes open. Bring and keep the chin on the chest, curve your shoulders forwards and downwards. To support yourself you will have the stirrup bars placed on each side of the bed. You will take a good hold of them and pull on them, spreading your elbows out slightly and keeping them slightly raised because they must not press on the bed. The pull you exert through the stirrup bars is not meant to bring the chest forward and to make you sit up on the bed, but it increases the curving of the neck and shoulders. You will repeat this exercise lying down, exactly as you will have to do it for labour, that is twice for one contraction. You will repeat it only once a week. On the other days, twice a day, you will lie on your bed and, after breathing in, blowing out, and stopping breathing, you will bring the chin on to the chest, so that you become familiar with the muscles which take part.

You must not breathe in and out twice in the second effort during a contraction. When the first effort is finished, you must breathe out and breathe in again, stop breathing, place the chin on the chest and begin pushing again. If you breathed twice, the contraction would be finished, and consequently you could not benefit from it.

This is all the work you have to do—added to the exercises you have already learnt. You are now in possession of all the essentials. It is up to you to use them as well as you can. Do not forget what you were told in the first lecture. Childbirth without pain is not childbirth without effort. You will have to make great efforts, and the better you are trained the better you will be able to make them.

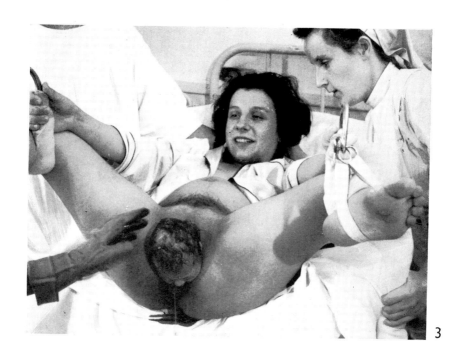

3

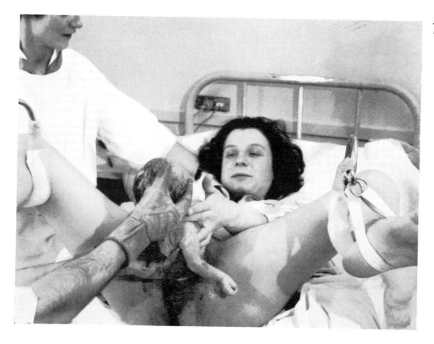

7

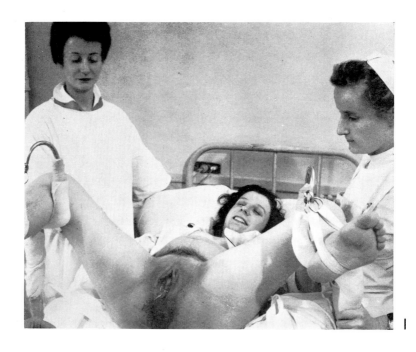

Mme. T. Para. 1. 24 years. Girl 5 lb. 11 oz. Conduct of labour: excellent

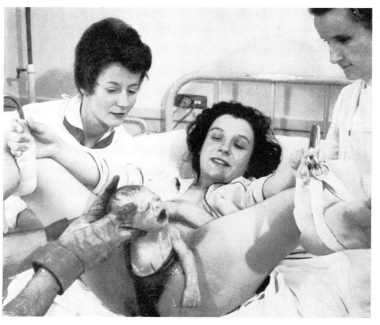

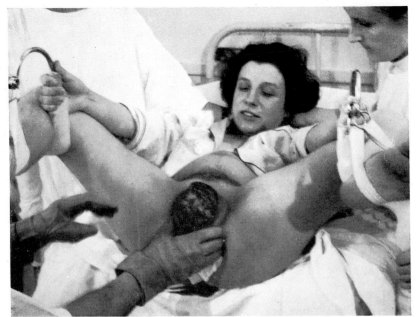

2

6

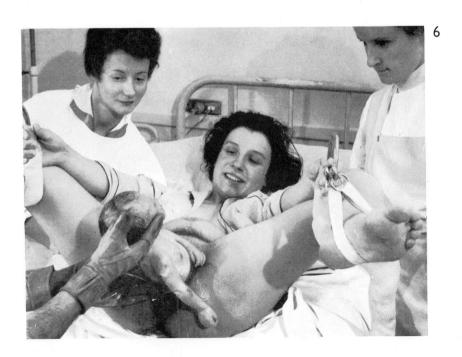

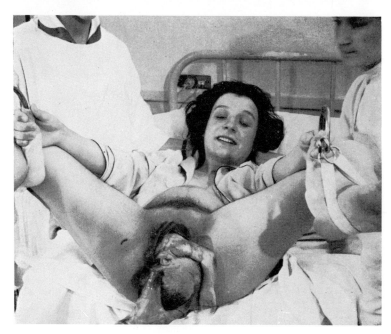

4

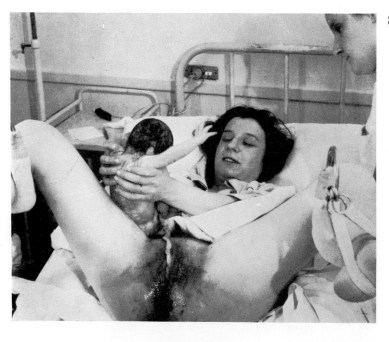

8

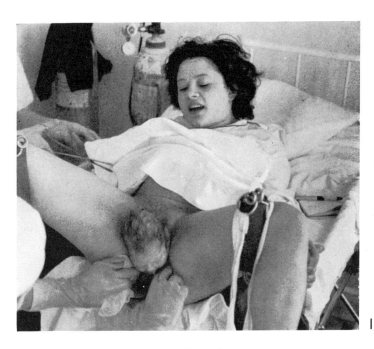

1

Mme. B. Para. 1. 20 years. Girl 6 lb. 14 oz.
Conduct of labour: excellent

2

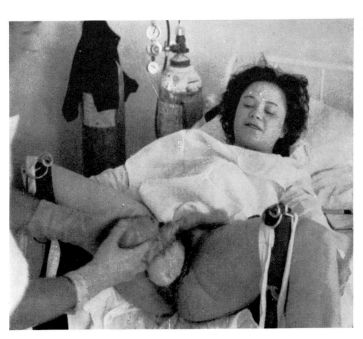

3

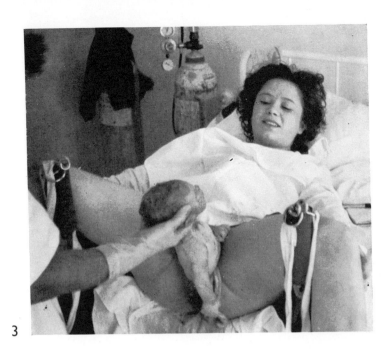

4

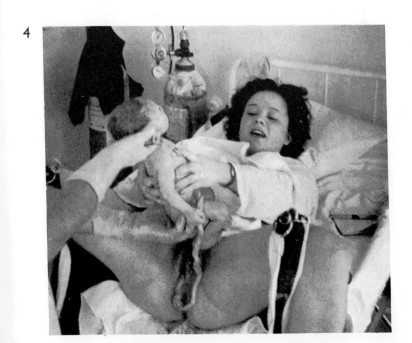

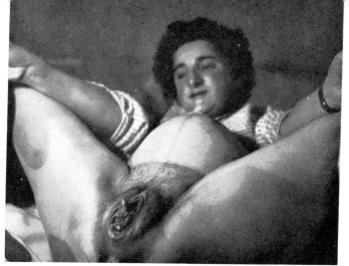

Mme. B.
Para. 2. 26 year
Girl 7 lb. 6 oz.
Conduct of
labour: excellen

1

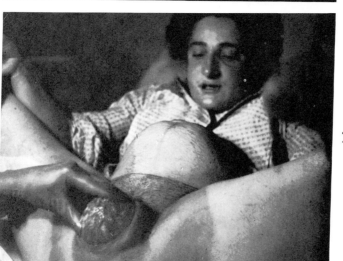

2

3

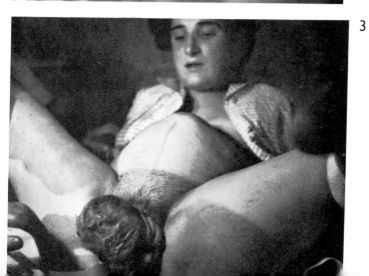

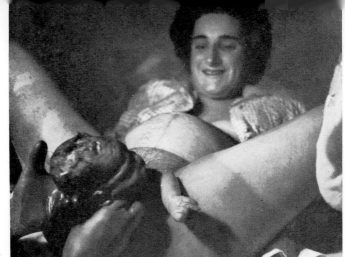

4

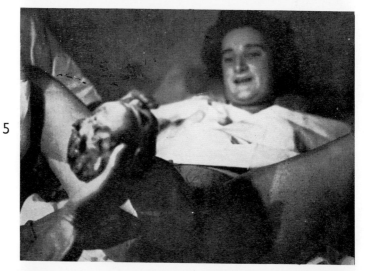

5

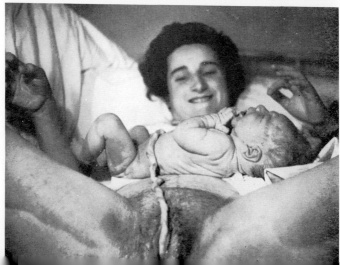

6

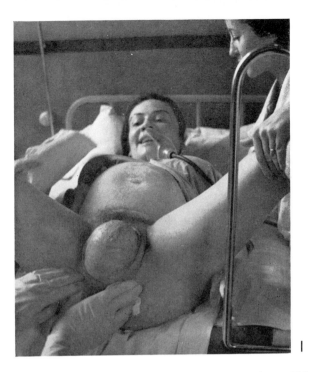
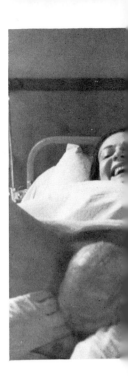

1

Mme. D. Para. 2. 23 years. Girl 7 lb. 14 oz. Conduct of labour: excellent

4

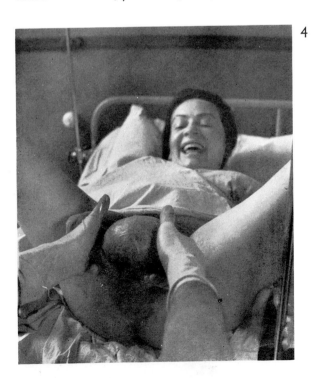
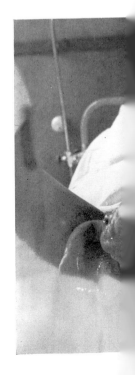

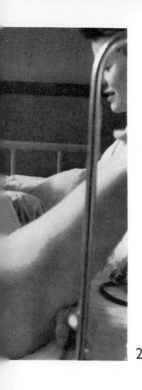

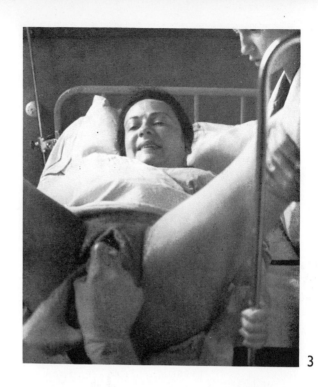

2

3

5

6

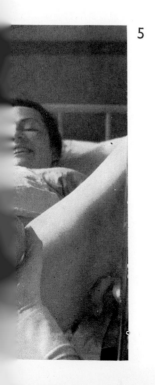

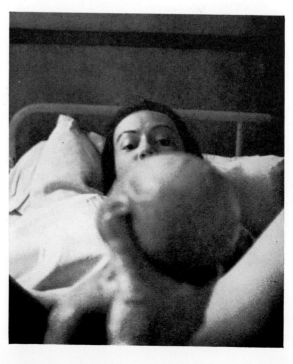

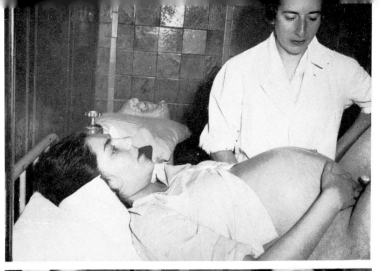

Mme. V.
Para. 2. 23 years.
Girl 8 lb. 10 oz.
Conduct of
labour: excellent

1

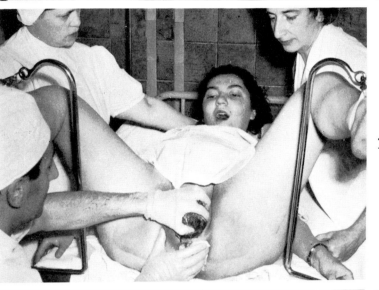

2

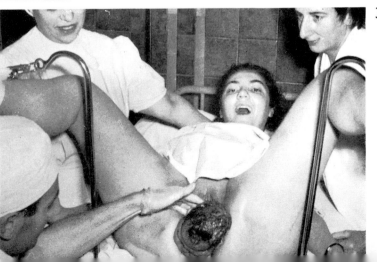

3

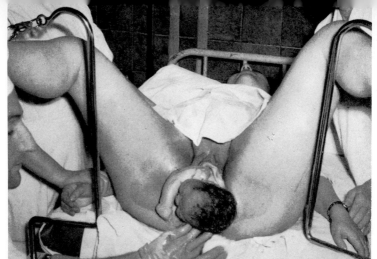

4

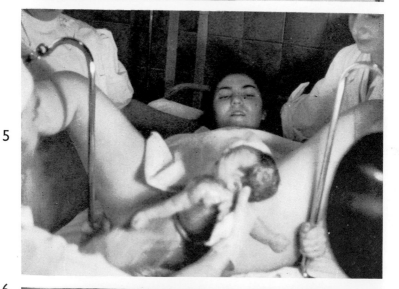

5

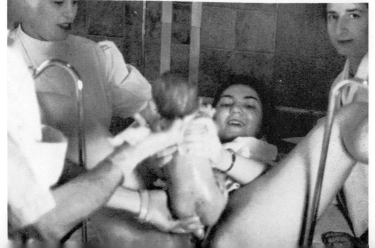

6

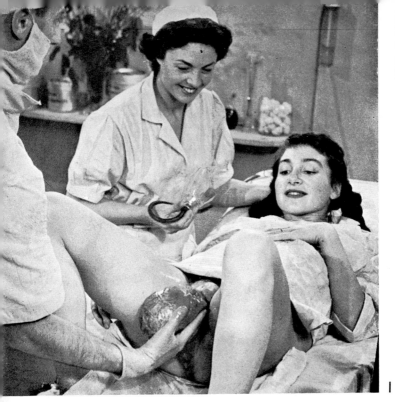

Mme. F.
Para. 2. 22 years.
Girl 7 lb. 11 oz.
Conduct of
labour: excellent

1

2

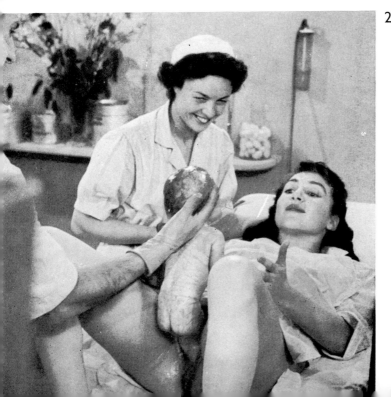

Photographs by Henry
Cohen from film on
childbirth without pain
produced by Fabiani,
Degliane and Dalmas.

Notes

THE last lecture interests the teacher as much as the woman. By now he should be able to judge what she knows, the practical use she has made of it and what she will be capable of doing with it.

The standard that the 'team' achieves depends on this final appraisal by the teacher. He should be able to predict events and leave nothing to chance. The study of the woman should be minutely carried out. It may involve a critical appreciation of the environment in which she lives. All this is not easy. The teacher is taught by his pupil. He learns all the time.

There is one question which we are often asked by doctors, midwives and others: 'Don't you get tired of always repeating the same thing?' It is a revealing question. From it we know that our questioner will not succeed in using the method.

No! We never repeat the same thing, although the rules remain identical. Each day we learn. What is there more varied than human beings? What is there more changeable than the environment in which the human being lives? Do you know of two identical women, of two identical teachers?

We are constantly enriched by the contact with human beings, and there is always something new, depending on the time, the place, the circumstances and ourselves.

When Dr. Lamaze was told, 'Out of thirty trained women, twenty failed,' he replied, 'Have you looked for the causes of *your* failures?'

In this last lecture, we emphasize that success is not only a question of confidence in the method or in the doctor or of belief or will-power. The brain is not the only factor in this success ('intellectual childbirth'). Neither is the practical side ('Develop your muscles in five lessons'). Nor does this success depend on a more or less mystical communion between the woman and the doctor.

Training for childbirth without pain by the psychoprophylactic method consists of an education where theory and practice are inseparable and have equal importance. Just as physiology—Pavlov teaches us this—is not cortical nor visceral: it is cortico-visceral.

Finally, the woman knows that labour can start in three different ways:

1. By the appearance of regular contractions.
2. By a loss of blood and mucus.
3. By the rupture of the membranes and loss of amniotic fluid.

She knows that, as soon as labour begins, she must 'respond' to a few contractions (shallow, quick respiration, relaxation, observation) in order to prove that contraction is accompanied by a normal and not painful sensation. She knows that she should go to the maternity home, if possible with her husband, as soon as she has clearly detected the first manifestations of labour. And she knows that she should leave home at the end of a contraction. Her training will then be finished. Success will depend on the use that she and the assistant make of what they have learned.

PART THREE

PERSONAL ACCOUNTS OF THE METHOD

Woman's Victory

THIS section is probably the most important and interesting in the book—moving evidence of woman's victory over herself. Our request to the women to write their impressions has been much criticized. People have said that such documents have no value—a curious judgment which would mean that a witness's evidence before a magistrate or a patient's report to a doctor is worthless. The women's reports seem to us important for various reasons:

1. They have given us doctors more information about the uterus in labour, the sensations that it transmits and its normal variations during labour; also about the sensitivity of the nervous system—towards interoceptors as well as exteroceptors.

2. They have stimulated and encouraged us in our difficulties, and have constantly proved that we were in the right. Some people have claimed that statements about childbirth without pain have been due to suggestion, but suggestion is not strong enough to make hundreds of women say they had no pain if they did, in fact, suffer.

3. The reports, in their simplicity, are encouraging to women who have not yet had children. Readers will derive comfort from them and look forward to their own successes. Childbirth without pain is an immense chain. Women are the links and their stories the solder.

4. Finally, these reports tell us a great deal about human beings. They reveal new possibilities. They are also warnings; we shall have to revise some of our ideas. We must question our patients and listen to them. This is the only way in which we can give them proper attention.

The reports are the most valuable human documents that we have ever had in our lives as doctors. All the women have given their written permission for us to publish them. Not one woman refused. They felt that they owed the method something, and this would help them to repay.

Psychoprophylaxis does not stop with childbirth; its influence goes on.

I

Primiparous Women

I N C.W.P. the primiparous woman has an advantage. She is going
through the experience for the first time. She has no difficult or
painful labour behind her which might make her say: 'Never
again.' Women in general who have difficult labour forget or think
they have forgotten. Then a new pregnancy comes along, and they
are continually apprehensive, thinking about the birth.

The primiparous woman has nothing like this to face, but she has
something to discourage her. Worst is a bad upbringing. In some
families childbirth goes well and in others badly. Where it goes well,
the idea of childbirth as a simple normal act is handed down from
mother to daughter, from generation to generation. But where it goes
badly each generation adds a little to the drama. At childbirth women's
powers of resistance are weakened.

A woman may be afraid of the society she lives in, and the fear will
reappear at pregnancy and in labour. She may have read unsuitable
books, which dramatize confinements, make them dreadful, and
imply that the mother is running a great risk.

The education of C.W.P. is at present given only to pregnant
women. They see—when they are prepared for the idea and have got
rid of all the mistaken stupid notions they have previously acquired—
that childbirth is a simple physiological act. In a few years these women
will tell different stories to their daughters. At present training is twofold. It has to do away with the influence of bad upbringing and then
to give a new rational education. In the next generation it will only be
necessary to complete the knowledge that the girl acquired in her
youth. What has been a great effort to the mother will be just an
ordinary effort for the daughter and perhaps very easy for the grand-
daughter.

At present the primiparous woman who indertakes training has to
clear her mind of mistaken teaching and then to attune herself. If she

is healthy and obstetrically normal, she can hope for a labour like those of the women here whose reports are almost hymns of joy.

NORMAL PRIMIPAROUS WOMEN

Mme Soizeau. Age: 29. Primip. 10 July, 1953. Boy 7 lb 4 oz

The doctor has asked me to write truthfully about childbirth without pain. I especially want to do this as I should like to encourage other women to avoid the much-too-easy way out of childbirth with anaesthetics.

At first I was somewhat sceptical, but little by little I was won over by the doctor's enthusiasm and deep conviction. He explained the basic principles of the method, and I had no more doubts. But then I wondered, 'Can I hold out?' I did hold out in spite of a few troubles—nausea, vomiting, backache.

Here are the details. On the evening of 9 July and morning of 10 July I noticed a slight discharge tinged with blood. I telephoned to the doctor who told me to see him in the afternoon and then to go to the nursing home. When he examined me he found that the cervix was completely taken up and one finger dilated. During the afternoon I felt no contractions, but had only backache, which returned at regular intervals—about every twenty minutes. I went to the nursing home between 9 and 10 p.m., and was taken to the labour ward at 10.30 p.m. At that time or soon afterwards I began to feel contractions about every fifteen minutes. They were quite weak and, to avoid tiring myself unnecessarily, I did not use quick breathing.

This phase lasted till 1.30 a.m., and then, during a much stronger contraction, I felt the membranes rupture. The midwife found that I was still only two fingers dilated. Then the contractions came more often and were stronger, and at about 2.30 a.m. I began quick breathing. I had to make an effort to detect the real starting point of a contraction and manage synchronization between contraction and quick respiration. Towards 3.30 a.m. the contractions came closer together and were stronger, and I felt that I was going to need the assistant who had trained me. She was summoned by telephone and arrived immediately. I cannot say what a comfort it is to have someone near you who is always calm and patient, maintains your morale and helps you physically—by massage.

At this time (two fingers to three quarters dilated) I felt two or three times what a contraction was like without quick respiration. I vomited during contractions and so could not breathe quickly. So I had the chance of comparison and can confirm the effectiveness of quick respiration combined with neuromuscular relaxation. I could remain completely relaxed only because Mlle G. massaged my loins during contractions.

In the last three hours of dilatation contractions came every three minutes and lasted about one minute. From time to time a longer contraction slipped in and lasted one and a half minutes, and this rhythm continued up to the end of dilatation. I knew from the periodic examinations that dilatation was progressing, and I waited for the urge to push which would show that delivery was starting.

But at no time did I have that feeling. Suddenly the contractions weakened and were more widely spaced and my backache disappeared. The doctor examined me and found that the baby's head was engaged in the upper canal. He decided that intravenous glucose was necessary to give me new muscular strength. A few minutes later I felt able to face the delivery.

This proceeded with a speed that astonished me. The doctor encouraged me by watching and talking, and I felt his co-operation, felt that I was no longer alone in pushing. So I produced the effort asked of me. I knew that in usual methods of childbirth the mask is put on when the baby reaches the perineum. So I imagined that the pain then must be almost unbearable. But pain in the strict sense did not occur. I felt a sensation of a great opening, but this did not reach the threshold of pain. In twenty minutes delivery was over and the baby had given his first cry.

This confinement, carried out by a method that respects the natural rules of childbirth, brought me twofold satisfaction. My baby suffered no injury or nervous shock and is in perfect health and very calm. And I experienced the indefinable happiness of having 'made' him—a complex feeling in which love, an instinct of possession and a certain pride were mixed. The first cry of my baby, which was a boy as I had wanted, is a wonderful memory.

Mme Trolonge. Age: 22. Primip. 13 November, 1955. Boy 6 lb 10 oz

Just before I found I was going to have a baby I heard of childbirth without pain from a friend who herself had recently had a little girl. It was a happy coincidence and I decided at once to adopt the new method.

Of course I was glad that childbirth could be without suffering.

But more than that I was attracted by the rational type of training. I like to know what awaits me and prepare myself. If there was any event in life which needed preparation it is surely the birth of a baby. Clear understanding, will-power and self-control can overcome bodily weakness and especially over-sensitive nerves and excessive imagination. 'The happy event', which has been accompanied in the past with anguish and screams, has become at last undiluted joy.

My delivery took place in complete happiness. Until then I had been entirely absorbed in controlling the contractions and resisting a desire to push. The work went on inside me; my part was only to control it. But now at last I could push, and the baby was going to be born.

And because I was becoming really active, I had the feeling that his arrival depended on me alone. It seemed that I was finishing his creation, helping in the completion of the work. My strength increased tenfold. I pushed six or seven times. I saw the head appear, the shoulders, and I had my baby placed on my stomach. It is an unforgettable moment, the greatest joy that a woman can know. My husband was beside me, trying to hide his tears. And then we were together and happy, admiring our work. Such memories can never be forgotten.

Mme du Raget. Age: 23. Primip. 6 August, 1953. Girl 7 lb 11 oz
. . . At about 12.30 a.m. the delivery began. The doctor gave me exact instructions and words of encouragement. He controlled and directed the movements I had to carry out to the smallest detail.

I was impatient to reach the end of these nine long months of waiting. I pushed as hard and as long as I could in the position taught during training. At each push the doctor announced the progress I had made.

In spite of an abnormal lie, my baby was brought on to my perineum by only seven contractions. I was very much afraid of the passage through the perineum—possibly through the fear of being torn and 'sewn together', an operation which had given me very unpleasant memories in my childhood. But here, as previously, the sensations were perfectly bearable —though I am generally pretty sensitive—and there was no tear.

The doctor showed me the head of my baby as it came out. I heard him say: 'The top of the head, the eyes, the nose, the mouth.' I pushed again, and he got a shoulder free, and then an arm, which he put on my stomach.

While my baby's head and chest were out, but her seat and legs still inside me, the doctor had to cut the cord, which was three times round her neck. I watched him do it, and did not feel any pain. During the whole of the last stage of childbirth I relaxed by practising quiet respiration with oxygen.

Then my little girl was born completely—a beautiful baby of 7 lb 11 ozs. This was at 1.30 p.m. The placenta followed a few minutes later, and again I felt absolutely no pain.

My confinement was exactly as it had been promised during the training. It was quick, well directed and ended well.

It followed a calm pregnancy without anxiety. I did not dread the moment when my baby should be born, and my life, behaviour and mood benefited throughout my pregnancy. I was surrounded by people who also believed in the method, and this helped me a great deal to maintain conviction, calmness and confidence. Also, the fact of knowing exactly how I was made—the position of my baby, what would happen when it came into the world, what I had to do at that moment—reassured me in the last months of waiting and prevented me from feeling any panic.

There were some factors which troubled me a bit at the clinic. Without these my confinement would have been still more satisfying. My usual assistant was on holiday. Her deputy, though very kind and full of solicitude—holding the oxygen mask for me and giving me fresh water-compresses on face and lips—had not the firmness of Mlle — who would not have let me slacken off for a second.

. . . I am now feeling marvellous and deliciously happy watching my little daughter in her cradle. I have the sensation of having achieved her birth in all ways, and I feel very proud.

Mme Longuet. Age: 32. Primip. 6 January, 1955
. . . The doctor helps you to detect the beginning and end of the contractions, but you get the idea quickly yourself. He encourages you while you push. At the time I realized more than usual the magic of the words which can take on the rhythm of the work to be done. Now I understand better the value and beauty of songs sung at work. They are a synchronization of breathing and the rhythm of the work.

Mme Zajdela. Primip. 11 October, 1954. Boy 6 lb 13 oz
The doctor has asked me to write a report on my confinement. I am also adding a few thoughts on 'pregnancy without worry'.

Childbirth had always seemed to me a terrifying thing, with its inescapable ending. When I became pregnant, I was distressed as well as joyful. On the advice of my sister-in-law, who had herself used the method, my husband and I decided to go and see Dr. V. I was not completely convinced at my first visit, but the doctor did succeed in saving me from that dull fear which seized me when I thought of what was going to happen to me. I understood that I must neither wait for the event nor submit passively but must go to meet it, to prepare for it to the best of my ability. 'You are going to train yourself,' the doctor said. 'You'll repeat your part hundreds of times, and when the day comes you'll know all that you have to do by heart. You'll control and not submit to your confinement.' This seemed impossible, but it was true.

In September, after six and a half months of unworried pregnancy, I began to train. Every day I did exercises. On four succeeding Mondays the doctor gave lectures which informed me on all the phases of pregnancy and confinement. Then Mme R. taught me the daily exercises, and the remaining worry was cleared up.

I felt that I was preparing for a very important rôle. I worked at it joyfully and energetically, and on the last day I had only one thought. I was to accomplish this wonderful act which would give me my baby.

On Monday, 11 October, when the first contractions began at about 4 a.m., I felt excited and proud. They were like my period pains. They came every ten or twelve minutes, and I began the quick superficial respiration and relaxed as much as possible. This was effective, and my husband and I stayed in bed till eight without worrying. Then I got up and went out to do my shopping. Whenever the contractions came, I turned to a wall and began to breathe—without worrying about the impression I was making.

Then I rang up Mme R., who advised me to go to the clinic for an examination in an hour's time. I went home. It was 9.30 a.m. I was so calm that my husband thought that the baby would not be born that day, and he went to see some urgent patients, promising to return as soon as possible to take me to the clinic. I blamed myself later for not going there by myself. If I had, I should have been able to relax, and the next few hours would have been easier.

Instead I stayed at home and found several small jobs still to be done—including my douche. My contractions were now coming every five or six minutes, and the smallest thing took quite a time to do.

When my husband returned at about 11.30 a.m., my cases were packed and I had made all my preparations, but I was far from relaxed and the contractions were becoming very painful. We left immediately for the clinic. It was noon. The midwife examined me and said that I was half dilated and that I should go at once to the labour ward.

The doctor was informed immediately as delivery, it was thought, would take place within an hour. In the labour ward I had one rather painful moment because I was told not to push. Quick respiration relieved me. Then the doctor arrived and my feet were put into the stirrups. What a wonderful moment. At last I was going to do something. I breathed in, blew out, stopped and pushed with all my strength —without worrying. Neither that first push nor the next four caused any pain. On the contrary, the perfect co-ordination between the contraction—to which I drew the doctor's attention as soon as it started—and the pushing, which he then asked me to do, suppressed all pain. Instead of being something to be feared, the contractions became a help. I waited for them; they brought me nearer to my baby's arrival. Then, in the middle of a push, the doctor told me to stop and breathe quickly. For two seconds I felt a cutting pain. Then I pushed again, and ten seconds later the doctor put my baby on my stomach.

I could not believe that it was over already. I was feeling perfectly well and able to appreciate intensely the extraordinary sensation of having a son born from me and because of me. The tenderness I felt was increased by the fact that I had been in control during the whole of this wonderful achievement.

What is more, I believe that it was not just a temporary experience. It is valuable to have worked out one's destiny in a constructive way. I now believe that one can excel oneself; can live each day to the full and control one's actions.

To be at last what I want to be. . . .

Mme R. Age: 24. Primip. 15 November, 1955. Girl 6 lb 10 oz

My little Josette is born. Now I have to do a more difficult job— write a report.

Young mothers who have not had the good fortune to experience childbirth without pain might find it unbelievable that writing *is* more difficult. But it is true in my case. Nature designed me to bring children into the world but not for a literary career.

I wanted to be a mother, and during the whole of my pregnancy

I was happy, in spite of the small troubles one has in this state. From the beginning we decided for childbirth without pain. I was, then, the perfect example of the mother-to-be—happy but ignorant. I expected a lot from this new method, although I knew nothing about it.

A small incident—detachment of the placenta—which occurred at the beginning of the seventh month nearly upset my hopes. But I recovered by a course of treatment which I followed whole-heartedly. I started my training three weeks before my confinement. The doctor encouraged me, or I should never have had complete confidence so near the end.

The first lecture was a revelation to me. At last I realized the importance of the work awaiting me and the happiness that would come through this work.

In two sessions I learned a great deal. I still fell short in many ways, but I had acquired enough assurance to carry out my task with the help of the doctor and assistant. Without them I should never have known how—or been able—to make a success of labour. I followed their advice—in complete confidence and with all my physical and moral strength. When the day arrived I had to go to the clinic suddenly, so that I was taken by surprise and went through some moments of anxiety as I waited for the assistant, though I had the comfort of my husband beside me. They were, of course, worrying moments for him too. To his great regret he had not been able to attend the doctor's lectures, and he had only heard of them through me.

What followed was too quick, and it absorbed me too much, for me to describe it all. As soon as the assistant arrived, I really began my work, and the doctor found me working hard and in good shape at the beginning of the final stage. Today it is very difficult to give my impressions. The experience was too great and beautiful. The moments were happy. I gave myself completely to the birth of our baby. Nothing is finer than to be able consciously to bring one's child into the world—without being prostrated by fear and pain.

The doctor, assistant and midwife were most helpful. My husband was there with his affection. I never felt alone, and I easily went through the last difficult minutes. With indescribable joy I received this small part of myself on my breast—the bond of our love. I shall always praise this method. Through it women can fulfil their natural function happily and fearlessly.

The opportunity of using it will certainly come again, and I shall not hesitate.

Mme Dominique Chautemps. Age: 24. Primip. 20 June, 1954. Girl 7 lb 11 oz

I was never afraid of my confinement, and every time I saw the doctor and Mme C. I grew more impatient for the day.

The doctor told me that I should probably give birth between 20 and 25 June. On the morning of the 20th I noticed I was losing a little blood and I felt something like period pains. In the intervals, which were of different length, I felt very well and active. I told myself that I need not think I had to give birth on that day just because the doctor had suggested the date. I thought I was imagining things, and decided not to take any notice of what I was feeling—since they were certainly not contractions. It seemed, from what I had learnt, that contractions had a definite start; that they came from the cervix and passed up over the whole uterus. My sensations were diffused. So I spent a very active day without doing the breathing or watching the time to see if the contractions were getting closer together.

At about eight o'clock I felt I must go home and lie down a bit and massage my stomach. Then everything went more quickly, and the contractions became more frequent. The first breathing exercises hardly helped me. I could not distinguish the beginning of the contraction and so start my respiration at the right time. Still, little by little the breathing—especially the quick breathing—and the gentle massage relieved my stomach pain. But I also had pain in the back and much greater pain in the thighs. At each contraction it was as if they were being gripped in a vice.

It was the most unpleasant moment of my confinement. My contractions seemed to be one long contraction, and I still believed that I was not yet in labour and that the birth would not occur for a day or two. But presently I got impatient and decided to go to the clinic for an examination to find out if labour had started. I arrived at 11.15 p.m., and was amazed to learn that I should be delivered in an hour. I was received very kindly and everything was all right. The doctor and Mme C. arrived, and I felt that we were all working together. After each push the doctor told me what progress I had made. Time did not count any more. I felt that everything was working by itself. At home it had been difficult to do the quick breathing. Here it began by itself and stopped by itself. I seemed not to have to interfere.

Until then, I saw, I had understood the lectures only theoretically. Now I felt completely impersonal and in the hands of a force as irresistible as the force that makes a tree grow. This may seem stupid, but it appeared a wonderful discovery at that time. I had no difficulty at all with the two moments which the doctor had said were the hardest for self-control.

I thought, with a little apprehension, that the head was about to come through. At the same second I felt my perineum grow numb. Then I heard the words, 'The eyes, the nose . . .' and then I pushed for the shoulder. I felt it warm and moist, and I looked and fully realized that I had a baby in my stomach and that it was coming out. At five to twelve my little daughter cried. I was so happy that I did not know what to do.

Back in my room I could not sleep. I felt as one does after a party. I wanted to relive all the moments which had passed too quickly.

I heard a woman groan, and the cries seemed to me absurd compared with my happiness.

Mme Lecouillard. Age: 40. Primip. 15 July, 1955. Girl 7 lb 6 oz

Primigravida at the age of forty! The prospect of motherhood would have filled me with fear if I had not had faith in the method of childbirth without pain. I was happy as I began my pregnancy and the long wait for the baby I wanted so much. I attended the lectures regularly and did my breathing exercises every day.

I had complete confidence in my doctor. I followed his advice exactly and my pregnancy continued with little trouble.

14 July, 1955. For two days, at intervals, I have felt my first contractions. As soon as they appeared I relaxed and breathed slowly, and easily avoided pain.

This morning they appear more distinct and closer together. At first they are every three hours, and then two hours. I have a heavy feeling at the base of my stomach and colic similar to that of my periods. As usual I get on with the housework.

10 o'clock. I go to market, walking more slowly than on previous days. I feel clearly that something is happening inside me. I stop walking at each contraction, but I still do not feel the need to start quick breathing.

1 o'clock. I have a good lunch with the family. But moving has become difficult, and I cannot walk too much. The contractions are more frequent, about every hour. During the afternoon I rest on the couch—alert, so that no detail escapes me.

4 o'clock. A relative comes to see me. For two hours I keep up bright conversation. I relax; breathe more quickly. The contractions disappear.

7.30 p.m. I prepare dinner, but I do not want to sit at the table, since from now on I shall have to do quick breathing. The contractions are coming every fifteen minutes. I go to bed at nine o'clock.

From 9 to 10.30 p.m. The contractions come more frequently— from every ten minutes to every five. I get up and dress calmly. My suitcase has been ready for several days. I have to go to the clinic in Paris—twelve and a half miles from Draveil. My husband gets the car out. It is 11.40 p.m. when we leave home. During the journey of half an hour I do the breathing with each contraction and control myself well.

Ten past twelve. We arrive at the clinic. I am examined by the midwife on duty. Dilatation is more than three fingers. The doctor and Mme C., the assistant, are called by telephone and arrive shortly afterwards.

One o'clock. I am now comfortably in position on the table. The assistant observes and regulates my breathing.

1.10 a.m. Examination and rupture of the membrane by the doctor. The baby is still high. I start the pushing stage. I observe the contractions carefully, so that I can work with them at the exact moment. The doctor advises me continually and corrects my position. I pull with all my strength on the stirrup bars, stop breathing and push strongly. I do it a dozen times. I am entirely absorbed. I have only one idea. My baby must not suffer and therefore should come through as quickly as possible.

The assistant keeps my face cool and encourages me. My husband, who has come with me to all the lectures, has wanted to be present. He helps me by his air of confidence.

1.50 a.m. I push out my baby's head. The labour is nearly over. I relax and breathe quickly for a few minutes again. Calmly the doctor describes my baby. It is a girl. Beatrice is born. It is 1.55 a.m. A few minutes later I learn her weight—7 lb 6 oz. Now I can indulge in my immense happiness. I have suffered nothing. I have only performed work which occasionally called for great effort. During the whole time I never felt that suffering was going to overwhelm me. I remember all the smiling faces looking at me. Beatrice's birth took place in a happy silence.

I am not tired. I can see admiration in my husband's look. He, too, feels he has taken part in this most moving experience—in which the word 'family' assumes its complete meaning.

All husbands should be present at their wives' confinements. Then they would cease to feel inferior, as they always do when they wait anxiously for the arrival of their children in the corridor of a clinic or outside the house.

And more and more mothers should insist on this psychoprophylactic method. It benefits themselves and also—and especially—their children.

Breech Delivery in a Primiparous Woman

Mme Poinet. Age: 31. Primip. 13 February, 1956. Girl 6 lb 10 oz

I was interested in the psychoprophylactic method before I was married. It seemed rational—both psychologically and physiologically.

To my joy I found that I was pregnant a few months after marriage. The only problem was to find a doctor who used this method. I had no prejudices to overcome, and so had an advantage over less well-informed mothers. I had an excellent pregnancy in perfect health with a quiet mind. I was very active. I camped, travelled by motor-bike, swam without trouble or fatigue. At the seventh month my baby's head was already in a good position and this indicated that confinement would be easy. Two days before birth it was a little high but well placed.

On Saturday, 11 February, I was awakened rather unpleasantly by a contraction. After the first surprise I calmed down, relaxed well and felt the next contraction less intensely. The contractions occurred every fifteen minutes. Was labour beginning? It seemed to me that the sensations should be stronger. The day passed, and I was busy as usual. At 7 p.m. the contractions were occurring every ten minutes, but they were still not very strong.

We were afraid that I should be kept at home by the ice and snow, so we left for the clinic. But labour had by no means started. I felt some contractions acting on the baby's head, which was still rather high. We went back home. In spite of the sedative suppositories which the midwife had prescribed, the contractions did not stop and I had to struggle to keep awake to note when each one started. They occurred now every five minutes, and the mucous plug came away.

We returned to the clinic at 12.30 p.m. on Sunday. Dilatation was still only just beginning. I went up to the labour ward. The rhythm of the contractions did not change till 10 p.m. Only their intensity increased. I kept my self-control well with relaxation and slow deep breathing. At 10 p.m. the midwife ruptured the membrane. The contractions became more frequent and I did the quick breathing. I still controlled myself well, but I felt very tired after two sleepless nights, and I was worried. Why did the midwives, who examined me in turn, say: 'The head won't engage,' and look a bit odd? I thought of various explanations. The cord might be too short. And I felt that dilatation would never end.

The doctor arrived. I was waiting impatiently for him. He told me that delivery was starting, and I was delighted. At last I was going to be active. Hope strengthened me, and I was not upset when I heard that it would be a breech birth. It was an extremely rare case. The baby had turned in the last forty hours. If I had known this I should not have been so impatient at the end of dilatation. I like an unpleasant truth more than even a slight doubt.

But the news was not really unpleasant, as I knew that childbirth without pain went very well even in the case of a breech. All I had to do was to push strongly. And here I must stress how necessary it is to prepare every day before childbirth. Every day I had scrupulously done my exercises, which my husband had firmly supervised. The first push had little effect because I did not carry out the doctor's orders properly. The reflex was faulty. But the next three pushes were sufficient. At 1.10 a.m. on the Monday I brought a little girl of 6 lb 10 oz into the world, and she had not suffered at all from her unusual birth. Without training I should have been one of those women who say: 'The pains went on for forty-five hours.'

I prepared myself for childbirth as I should for an examination. I thought about it very often. I studied it, I must confess, more with intellectual curiosity than maternal feeling. I wanted to succeed for the baby's sake and my own, but I also wanted to overcome my friends' doubts. The woman who is fortunate enough to give birth happily feels it her duty to let others benefit from her experience. The more women want childbirth without pain, the more quickly will the authorities have to take steps to spread the method. And it is being recognized that it is not just the ungodly invention of materialistic scientists, but has human value. It suppresses the pain of course, but—more important—it keeps the mother fully conscious and dignified and allows her to experience unforgettable moments of emotion.

The doctors who train her are more than doctors. They are teachers who help women as personalities to become conscious of themselves.

Forceps Delivery Without Anaesthesia

Mme Quentin. Age: 37. Primip. 6 January, 1955. Girl 6 lb 10 oz

Here I am a few days after coming home—happy. I have brought back my pretty little girl—exactly what I wanted—and I had no pain. It is wonderful. I keep on going to see if the cradle is still there and it is not a dream. Yet I shall never forget that 'happy event'. It was well worth while giving a few minutes morning and evening to the training. Our little co-actors are willing to play their parts only on the day of the show, and they know their own rôles perfectly. It is up to us not to miss a cue, and then all will go well.

On Thursday, 6 January, at 3.30 a.m., I had the first warning—a watery discharge. I got up, trying not to wake my husband—as the doctor has advised in the last lecture. But back in the bedroom I found him beginning to dress. I had the greatest difficulty in making him return to bed—and myself too. He wanted to take me to the clinic. It seemed funny to see him in such a panic. I have never laughed so much. But I had explained to him what we had been taught.

I left for the clinic at two o'clock when the contractions were occurring every quarter of an hour. The assistant came to me, and the first phase passed very well.

The next stage was not so happy. We had been taught that we should want to push. But I did not want to. I felt as though the baby were pushing and I had to hold back. I felt like a ship that wants to drop anchor in port where there is room for a fishing boat only.

Twice I almost sank. Fortunately, Mme C. was there, and, thanks to her, I got my breath back. Then I started again—this time without a hitch.

I hardly dare to speak of the delivery. The doctor did all the work. He used two big spoons that looked like a fruit-salad server. Then I pushed and he managed to catch my baby. It is wonderful and moving to see the doctor make your baby come into the world, give it to you and say whether it is a boy or girl. And that is all.

No, not all. Thanks to the relaxation method that was taught me I am curing my worst fault—losing my temper. When I get worked up and feel as if I am going to explode, I find a quiet corner and relax. The temper goes only gradually—but it goes. Now that I am a mother

I do not want my husband to call me a tigress as he used to. I should be ashamed in front of my daughter.

Thank you, doctor. Through you we are going to be still happier than before.

Mme Cohen. Age: 24. Primip. 14 February, 1955. Boy

. . . The doctor put on the first and then the second half of the forceps. The second was a bit painful, but only for a very short time. I still wanted to push. I pushed while the doctor pulled the baby, and I did not feel the instruments at all. Nor did I feel the episiotomy. The doctor told me to rest a little. Then I pushed a bit more to help him free the shoulder. I saw my husband opposite me looking at his baby— and I saw my son. He was put on my stomach.

It is difficult to describe my feelings. I do not know what to say. He was there. I looked at him. He cried.

I owe all this to the method. Not only did I not suffer, but I experienced this moment. In spite of the forceps I was not anaesthetized. I had no pain and I saw my baby come.

Mme F. Age: 18. Primip. 1 April, 1955. Boy 8 lb 6 oz

. . . In spite of difficulties I have no regrets. Thanks to the psychoprophylactic method I have had the proud joy of giving birth to my baby and one of the most wonderful moments of my life. At no time did I feel the least anxiety. I avoided a Caesarian and even an episiotomy through co-operating with the doctor, and I had forceps without anaesthesia. So I have proved to my family and friends that childbirth without pain is not something to be laughed at.

Dr. Georges de Werra, previously obstetric registrar, 4, Place Pepinet, Lausanne, writes of forceps without anaesthesia:

. . . On the evening of my return from the congress, I had the opportunity of using forceps without narcosis. This is what the woman wrote in her report:

'It is an extraordinary thing to take part in the birth of one's baby in this way. I should not have forgiven the doctor if he had anaesthetized me at the end—even for the use of forceps. I should have felt cheated of the essence of this adventure, like a mountaineer whose eyes are bandaged when he has a wonderful view before him after making great efforts.'

2

Multiparous Women

HERE two different categories must be noted:
    1. Those who have had one or more normal deliveries. To use their own words they 'had pain, of course, but *nothing more*' and now have no very unpleasant memories.
    2. Those who have had difficult—sometimes dreadful—deliveries. These women have terrible memories.

The first category is very similar to the primiparous women. Good training and their own desire to succeed will produce a completely satisfactory childbirth, though the actual delivery of the baby may be more difficult than with the primigravida, for they have suffered some damage from their previous confinements.

The second category forms one of the great problems of childbirth without pain. A powerful signal has to occur only once to create a definite conditioned reflex. A bad delivery acts in this way, and it will be difficult for the teacher to destroy the reflex thus created. He will succeed, however, if the woman will co-operate sufficiently. The woman herself may quite understand her difficulties at the first birth and her chance of success now if she is trained; but a doubt may persist which will handicap her and lead to only partial success.

But this partial success will be valuable. It may be imperfect, but it will get rid of the memory and inhibiting influence of the first childbirth for ever. The woman finds herself freed, as it were, and this alone is a very great achievement. Hundreds of women, who have had previous children, have told us, radiant with joy, 'For the first time I have managed to bring my baby into the world by myself. . . . To think that I didn't have the experience before and didn't want to believe that it could happen.'

Any woman who will conscientiously try the method can prove its value.

Mme D. Age: 24. Para. 2. 26 October, 1954. Boy 9 lb 14 oz

It was at the end of a very tiring day, when I was weary and my nerves were on edge, that I felt the first contractions coming every twenty minutes. I realized that I was extremely well conditioned, for my tiredness and nerviness completely disappeared when I found that my labour had started. I immediately felt in a very good mood, though a little excited and nervous like an actor before a performance. I had a bit of stage-fright. But I was really in a state of well-being when I crossed Paris to go to the clinic, and the city had never seemed so beautiful to me.

When the midwife examined me, I was two fingers dilated. I immediately started to relax, and found it very easy. From that moment I ceased even to be afraid that I should spoil my delivery. I felt that it would be very simple.

While I was waiting for Mme R., my assistant, I reread the accounts of confinements at the end of Colette Jeanson's book. I wanted to try the respiration, but there was no need. Because of my relaxation I was simply not feeling the contractions. I went very quickly from two to three fingers.

The relaxation was the exact opposite of what I had achieved by a great effort of will in the first stage of my confinement three years before. I had read Dr. Read's books at the time and had resolved not to suffer; but that was not enough by a long way. I screwed myself up in the effort to relax, but I did have pain and the unpleasant feeling all the time of being on the point of giving way and screaming. But this time relaxation needed no effort. It was inside me, and I should have had to make a great effort to scream and an even greater effort to have pain.

But—contrary to what a woman should feel in a second childbirth without pain—I felt very dependent on Mme R. and the doctor, and was glad to see them arrive.

The doctor ruptured the membranes, which I did not feel, but immediately the contractions became stronger and more frequent. It was the beginning of the difficult phase. It is only at this time, I think, when one is half to three quarters dilated, that the respiration becomes necessary. I did it with Mme R., and this prevented me from getting out of breath. But I was very tired—it was three o'clock in the morning —and my eyes closed between the contractions. Several times at the end of a contraction I almost fell asleep, and I was woken up by violent pain which was a new contraction beginning. Immediately I practised the respiration, and what I had felt as pain when half asleep became simply a violent muscular sensation—and yet the contraction was at its height. There are obviously clinical and mechanical reasons why the breathing has this effect, but what I felt strongly at that moment was that I was changing from a passive person while I was half-asleep to an active person controlling the contraction instead of giving way to it. The danger of this phase of strong contractions is, I think, of feeling oneself passively carried away. That was why Mme R. was so useful at the time—warning me that a contraction was beginning, helping me to regulate my breathing, explaining exactly what was happening and applying cold water to refresh and wake me up.

One is very selfish at this time, and the conversation of the doctor, my mother-in-law and my husband began to disturb me. I think I wanted everybody to concentrate on me and my childbirth, and I was happy when they left me alone with Mme R. This difficult phase lasted only a short time—twenty minutes. I felt the first desire to push. Fortunately Mme R. was there to remind me to do the quick respiration. I had completely forgotten.

Things happened very quickly. There was just time for the doctor to put on his gloves, and the delivery really started. I pushed with a feeling of great relief and even of pleasure. At last I could be intensely active. Yet I did not push very well. I could have delivered the baby in three pushes, and it took me five. It was not because I was afraid of being torn or having pain. These things did not cross my mind. But there was some misunderstanding when the head reached the perineum. I let my breath go, and then I waited for the doctor to tell me to push. He, I think, was waiting for me to indicate a contraction. In the end I had absolutely no pain, and I pushed very hard, and it was a very satisfying moment when I felt the baby moving through me. I did not even realize when the head passed, but I think I shall remember all my life the sensation of sweetness and warmth which the baby's body gives as it comes out. The sensation lasts for only a second, but from that moment I felt the child to be mine. Perhaps I have shocked some people by describing this feeling in detail. But it was the climax of my childbirth, and I often think of it now when I am attending to the child. It is also really the end of labour.

The doctor put the baby on my stomach and he cried immediately. I was expecting to be very moved and to cry too. I was certainly very moved, but I did not want to cry. I laughed instead.

I remember how I woke up from my first confinement—crying

and incapable of taking any interest in the baby, who was already dressed and in a corner. My first thought when I saw him was: 'Why have they brought a baby here?' So little did he seem to belong to me.

This time the doctor pulled gently on the cord, and the placenta came away immediately. The baby was very big—9 lb 14 oz—and tore me a little. This would not have happened, but I already had a scar, and one stitch must have given way. The doctor repaired the damage immediately without an anaesthetic. It felt like the prick of a pin.

In a second childbirth without pain, I think, one should be able to appreciate what is happening inside oneself better. In fact I had a feeling, once childbirth was finished, of not having completely taken advantage of the situation. I had been so busy with the breathing and then the pushing, and everything went so quickly. The delivery lasted only three to five minutes. It is somewhat like a violent effort made in mountain-climbing; there is no time to look at the view. I really had no time to think about what I felt. That is my only disappointment.

To have made a success of childbirth leaves you with a feeling of very great contentment—almost of superiority. I lived the last month before the birth constantly thinking about it, imagining it exactly as I wanted it to happen, carrying Colette Jeanson's book with me everywhere like a talisman, and attaching great importance to the doctor's and assistant's lectures. I probably bored my friends and relations very much by constantly talking about it. But this was all good conditioning and helped me to succeed. This serious approach is certainly necessary—at least during the last months—even if ironic remarks are made, as they always are. As well as the experience itself of childbirth without pain, which is moving and beautiful, one finds oneself afterwards with entirely new reserves of strength and calmness. With me this was manifested in a rather odd way. I have completely stopped biting my nails—which I have been doing since childhood. This really is a noticeable result!

Mme Jaeger. Age: 24. Para. 16 March, 1955
Childbirth without pain should, it seems, be a conscious experience rather than a means of avoiding suffering. I came to it with an unpleasant memory of a difficult first confinement. I had been overcome with pain, had begged for an anaesthetic and had thought that I should die.

I am a dancer. For many years I attempted to dominate my body, control my muscles and liberate it by relaxation—which I practised for two years. And now I very much wanted, through this childbirth, to work in the same way—to achieve a synthesis of myself as an artist, woman and mother.

From the first—with everybody talking so simply of the end of pregnancy—I trusted this method. It was so similar to the one I had used as self-expression. During the long months in normal conditions, the fruit ripened. It had to fall normally and continue its autonomous existence.

When one morning I found myself in bed at the clinic, I was not anxious. I was happy to bring my labour into time with my breathing. As I went from two fingers to half dilatation, my mind rose above the waves of pain. In the last phase it was sometimes difficult to keep myself under control, but each victory over the stronger and stronger contractions made me still more careful and contented. My assistant was a most effective help in these moments. On the table the intense mental tension was replaced by an almost entirely physical effort, and I felt great relief. I was in action. I took part directly. My mind strained towards the birth. Neither time, pain, nor the fatigue of my arms mattered. The doctor directed my energies. I drew moral strength from the midwife's attention and my husband's clasp on my hand. And so I went forward to delivery. The first cry was the final stage of the adventure. I feel proud of it and happy.

At no time did I lose control of my mind. Nor did I relive the nightmare of my first confinement. And so I have every reason to be satisfied with the method. What is more, I found a confirmation of my philosophy of life in it—a direct relationship with my work of dancing as I had evolved it after years of research.

I still do the breathing exercises, and they and the new understanding of how to renew energy will remain a permanent acquisition. I shall try to put them to practical use.

And now I am happy and free and healthy in a way that astonishes me.

Mme C. Age: 28. Para. 2. 22 June, 1955. Girl 7 lb 15 oz

My report would have no significance unless I said something about the great handicap from which I suffered—the memory of my first confinement. I did not, of course, suffer more than others. I had fifteen hours of labour, forceps, three stitches. It was a childbirth similar to many others. But for many months I was obsessed by the memories of those tortures which are cynically called 'a happy event'. I was revolted. It seemed to me that a monstrous error had lasted for centuries. When I read a report about 'childbirth without pain', I felt that at last doctors had understood, and I agreed to have a second baby.

But in spite of the good intentions with which I set about training, I never managed to get rid of my fear completely.

I had many contractions at the end of pregnancy. They were painless in the daytime, but woke me up at night in a very unpleasant way. Several times they became regular and frequent (ten minutes; then seven minutes), and I thought I ought to leave for the clinic. I waited for them to get stronger, but instead they became less frequent and stopped after a few hours.

At last, on the night of the 22nd, fifteen days before the expected date, I was woken up at about five o'clock by contractions like the ones I had felt so often. I did not worry much, and tried to go back to sleep. But they rapidly became stronger, and I realized that this time it was the real thing. So I got ready to leave—a bit nervous but very happy. I did my rapid respiration, more for practice than from necessity.

When I arrived at the clinic, to my surprise the midwife who examined me said that I was already three fingers dilated. It was about 7.30 a.m.

The doctor came a little later. Labour had not progressed, and he gave me an injection of sparteine to speed things up. After the injection the contractions became strong and almost continuous. I could not afford to breathe normally any more. I breathed as quickly as possible—not always very brilliantly.

I cannot say that I had no pain at all. But these pains remained easily bearable until the end of dilatation, and could not be compared with the pains I had the previous time.

Then delivery began. And I really was afraid.

No doubt because of that—and contrary to what younger mothers say—this final stage seemed to me more difficult. I did the first push timidly and unwillingly. It hurt me.

I felt this was because I was not giving myself completely, and was also not controlling myself well. The next time I did better; the third, too. I cannot remember how many times I pushed—perhaps four or five. I only know that it stopped being painful when I had the courage to push as hard as I could.

The head passed quickly and without difficulty. I was then told to relax before the delivery of the shoulders. This was the most difficult moment of the whole labour. My courage gave way. I was not even brave enough to look at my baby, whom I could already have seen.

At last the arms were freed. A moment later my daughter was put on to my stomach. She was wonderful. I was overcome with joy.

It was 9.40 a.m.

When the doctor said, 'Now, was it worth the trouble?' I replied 'Yes.'

Very sincerely.

Mme R. B. Age: 30. Para. 5. 20 July, 1954. Girl

I have never been afraid of a confinement. The first time I suffered for a whole night and had only a vague idea of what was happening. But my unpleasant impressions vanished as soon as the baby was born.

The second time I had a big dose of pituitary, and they gave me chloroform. It was all over in half an hour, but I have an evil memory of the contractions after the pituitary injection.

The third and fourth confinements were conducted much better, and I did not suffer at all. But this was because of artificial means—a small amount of pituitary, a light anaesthetic during dilatation, forceps and general anaesthesia at the end. When I woke up they brought me the baby bound up and slightly bruised.

I was interested in childbirth without pain as soon as people began to talk about it. There were lectures, films, articles and reports of friends—which impressed me especially when they had had children before, as then they could make comparisons between their child-births. When I was pregnant again, for the sake of the baby and my curiosity I tried the experiment.

Today, a few days after the birth of my little girl, I realize that everything was better than I had hoped. Not only is the child pink and undamaged, calm and healthy, but I am feeling other benefits. I am absolutely relaxed and peaceful, and I have had practically none of the post-natal pains from which I suffered abominably on previous occasions.

Morally I have the satisfaction of having kept myself under control —thanks to the training—and self-mastery is always an uplifting feeling. For the five hours of dilatation I was perfectly conscious of the need for control. I did not suffer at all. Suffering implies inactivity, and there was not a single moment of this. Even at the beginning of the contractions, when one has to relax, all one's attentions must be concentrated on this dilatation, and one must try to follow its progress.

I felt that quick respiration was necessary when my contractions became stronger. But I was only two fingers dilated, and after an hour it was still the same, However, less than twenty minutes later I said to my assistant that I had made a lot of progress. She called the midwife, and I was in fact half-dilated.

I have already said that I was in no pain, but I felt that I rose above the pain as an airman flies above a mountain, and that, if my engine failed for lack of petrol, I should run into it violently.

Delivery lasted five minutes. I marked time unnecessarily, it seemed, before pushing. The doctor explained that this was because of my previous confinement which had ended with forceps. I was at a stage where I had got into the habit of letting myself go.

Finally, as a last act the baby was put on my stomach before the cord was out. I was the first to see, touch and know it. At that moment I completely lost control. It was my fifth daughter. I should have liked a boy. But I was so happy to have this baby, which seemed so much my own, that I laughed foolishly from joy and tenderness without being able to stop.

Mme Dreyfus-Gauthier. Age: 35. Para. 4. 10 June, 1954. Twin girls 5 lb 8 oz and 5 lb 1 oz

On the evening of Wednesday, 9 June, while I was doing my housework, I felt the pain in my back get worse. It had started the night before. I had difficulty in moving my right leg, and this lasted until the delivery of the second baby, who must have pushed on a nerve centre.

I went to bed at 10.30 p.m. I had a few contractions, but I made sure that they were not regular and did not worry any more. I relaxed, breathed deeply, and went to sleep at about eleven. At 12.30 a.m. I awoke and noticed that I was losing some blood. So I was sure labour had started. I woke my husband so that he could help me get ready. The birth was not expected until the end of June. I had to shave myself and carry out all the doctor's instructions. We did this scrupulously, dressed, telephoned the clinic to say we were coming and arrived about 4.15 a.m. The contractions continued, but they were irregular. I went on with the deep breathing and had no pain. As soon as I arrived the midwife examined me, and found I was three fingers dilated. She called for my assistant and the doctor. Mme D. arrived half an hour later, and the doctor soon afterwards. Meanwhile the midwife had given me an injection to relax the cervix. The first baby was pressing on the front of the cervix, which was not taken up.

Meanwhile the contractions were coming more often and had become more regular. I admit that sometimes near the end I could not keep up my quick breathing. I had exceptionally long contractions, and I had missed three weeks of training. But Mme D. reprimanded me when I stopped trying. She reminded me to relax and softly stroked my stomach, which also helped.

The doctor gave me an injection of coramine glucose to sustain my heart, and my husband gave me the oxygen mask.

At 6.30 a.m. I was fully dilated and I was put into position for delivery. This stage seemed to me to pass very quickly and I was quite surprised when my husband told me it had lasted twenty minutes. My first daughter was born at 6.50 a.m. I can remember the doctor's voice. It was a strong stimulus. I kept up the last push—which really delivered the baby—because I heard him say: 'Don't give way. You're there,' and in fact I was.

Then they let me rest ten minutes. The doctor took the opportunity to turn the second baby, who, with more space, had moved completely across. With a skill for which I am infinitely grateful, he brought the head into a good position and ruptured the second membrane. At the same time I had a small dose of pituitary, since the uterus was tired and could not contract and the doctor felt the cervix hardening already. Immediately the contractions began again. I pushed during two contractions, holding my breath two or three times as I was told to do. (The midwife helped me in the first one by pushing on the fundus of the uterus.) I delivered my second little girl, with two contractions, at 7.10 a.m.

I cannot say that I did not suffer at all as I had pain in my back, but we were told that at present this cannot be relieved. But I know what the ordinary childbirth is like, so that I can say how effective the new method is. Although my perineum is in a bad state, this time I had no tear.

This childbirth is my fourth. The first two were catastrophic. The first baby had a hemiplegia at birth, and the second was suffocated and still-born. The third was almost normal, but the delivery took place without an anaesthetic, and once more I was cut and sewn up.

This time I could consciously see my two babies coming into the world, hear their first cries and feel the comforting warmth of the little bodies through the towel that was put on me. I could actually take part in the birth of my daughters.

It is five days since my delivery, and I can get up without feeling tired, walk about my room, move without effort and above all feed the babies. It is the first time that I have had enough milk to half-feed my two babies, which means that I could feed one completely, and I am amazed at this.

It would not be nearly enough merely to thank the doctor and his assistant. The task these teams carry out is enormously important. At last the woman who brings a baby into the world is considered something more than a beast of burden. She is no longer left with her pains, not understanding why such a natural event can be such torture.

I hope that units specializing in the new method will be set up in French hospitals.

Mme M. Age: 30. Para. 2. 23 May, 1955. Girl 8 lb 2 oz. Breech

At your suggestion I am sending an account of my confinement.

I had been on the alert for a few days, because when I last saw you I knew I should not have long to wait.

On Sunday, the 22nd, at about 10 a.m., I felt the first symptoms. My husband was with me from the start, and that kept me calm. Until one o'clock I carried on as normally as possible. I had small contractions about every ten minutes, but I got over them easily by slow deep breathing. Suddenly I felt I wanted to pass urine and the waters came away in a jet. From that moment everything happened quickly. The contractions became more violent and intense, and I thought it was time to go to the clinic. I set off, trying to use the quick superficial respiration as well as I could. I felt a bit lost, especially as I knew I was going to have a breech delivery.

As soon as I arrived at the clinic, at 2.30 p.m., I was taken to the labour ward. I was half dilated and my cervix was soft. Everything was going well. I calmed down. My assistant helped and encouraged me at weak moments, and everything went very well. About 3.15 p.m. you, the doctor, arrived. I felt the need to push immediately, and at 3.50 p.m. my daughter was born, without any tearing, in a peaceful relaxed atmosphere.

My husband and I were amazed at the results of childbirth without pain. I could never have imagined such success. There is no comparison with ordinary childbirth—which I remember from the birth of my son.

The success, from my point of view, goes back to the consultation in the seventh month of my pregnancy. I learnt that I had gained too much weight (9 to 11 lb in one month) and that I should have a breech delivery. I was demoralized when I left you, doctor. I must be frank with you. I said to myself, 'You've begun to gain too much weight again, and you're going to have a breech, That isn't a very good start, my dear.'

And yet it was the beginning of victory for me. I felt the urge to take charge of the situation, to gain control of myself again. I exactly followed the diet you prescribed. It worked, and I lost 4½ lb in eight days. This encouraged me, and I regained my physical and moral equilibrium. Everything seemed easy. I was relaxed. Then came the theoretical and practical classes. I did the exercises and the quick shallow breathing every day to give myself the best chance. And so I faced up to childbirth.

I should like to tell all future mothers using childbirth without pain that they must not be discouraged if they have moments of weakness. They will make a success of childbirth according to their self-control and confidence in their doctors and assistants. Here lies the key to the mystery. I want to thank you, doctor, especially as you showed me this.

Mme T. Age: 32. Para. 3. 5 January, 1954. Boy 10 lb 1 oz. Forceps delivery

Here I am at last with my aim achieved. I have brought my third baby into the world.

When I was waiting for my first baby I cried with disappointment, I remember, because everything was going to happen without my husband and myself taking part, and neither of us would hear the first cry of our first-born. I tried to discuss it with the doctor, but he was doubtful and gently ironic. 'We'll discuss it again,' he said, 'when you're three fingers dilated.' But when the time arrived, I was exhausted after a very long dilatation which ended with forceps, and I did not think of refusing the anaesthetic. My husband, who had not left me for a day and a night, was sent to walk up and down the corridor, and he has only just forgotten the misery of that confinement.

Two years later, when my daughter was born, I did not dare to ask for delivery without an anaesthetic. Dilatation was much quicker. The baby was smaller. And during my stay at the clinic I went through a period of depression. I told myself that I could easily have reached the end of childbirth by myself, but like a coward I had let myself be deprived of this joy. I remember a feeling of failure, shame and frustration, and I could not get rid of it.

It was only during my third pregnancy that I heard of childbirth without pain. I was much relieved after my first interview with the doctor. He, like me, was convinced that it is normal for a woman to want to take part in the birth of her baby. With him there was no question of masochism, female curiosity, self-punishment or any other sinister interpretation which my queries had aroused. I should say that it was not so much the words 'without pain' that attracted me but finding a doctor who backed me up in my wish to take part in the delivery. From now on I began to look forward to my confinement.

And now the confinement. At three o'clock in the morning I was suddenly taken with strong frequent pains. I had to dress and close my case hurriedly while I was trying to do the quick respiration. The effect was dubious. It was only when I reached the clinic that I could relax and regulate my breathing, and immediately all went well. I not only did not suffer, but I felt surprisingly calm, happy and confident. This complete absence of fear seemed the chief feature of the confinement. I was warned at the end of dilatation that the pains would grow stronger. But I was surprised to feel them as pure sensations which were not painful. I controlled them more and more easily.

Then came the delivery. I could not believe that I was going to feel my baby coming out of me. From the first push I noticed that the pain was completely neutralized if I stopped breathing and bent my head forward. Unfortunately the baby was very big and badly rotated. The doctor told me that he was going to help it with forceps. This did not frighten me at all—thanks to a report I had read by a young woman recently delivered in the same conditions, who said she felt no pain. I relaxed completely, and felt nothing when the forceps were introduced. Only the stretching of the perineum seemed painful— probably because it recalled my first confinement when I woke up under the anaesthetic and for a few seconds felt a pain which it took me a long time to forget.

Thanks to the forceps I felt relief immediately, knowing that the head was coming through and I was no longer pushing in vain. And then there was the joy—impossible to describe—of feeling the little limbs slip through and having my son on my stomach when he gave his first cry, with my husband there as happy and calm as myself.

The only difficulty I had during the birth was to stop myself thinking of my first delivery. I felt that if I did not try my hardest to forget it, I should give way. At my first confinement I felt I was drifting on a stormy sea. This time I felt that I had learned to steer and ride the waves. From now on it lay with me whether I reached port or took in water and capsized. It seems to me now that the emotional and therapeutic value of the method lies to a large extent in this struggle against pain to give birth joyfully.

3

Women who have already experienced
Childbirth Without Pain

M ANY women have already experienced childbirth without
pain two or even three times.

One experience is not enough to enable a woman to
repeat the process without further conditioning. The training from the
first occasion is too fugitive. Childbirth without pain is not an easy
answer. We have seen women doing extremely well at their first
confinement but not so well at the second—because they were too
sure of themselves and neglected their training.

On the other hand those who train seriously for each confinement
steadily improve their achievement. One woman wrote: 'The first
time it was as if I were on a tight-rope. The second time I felt I was on
the road. The third time it was as if I were in the Champs-Elysées.'

Possibly by the fourth or fifth childbirth without pain the woman
will have acquired a cortical equilibrium and the right response, and
will be able to do without any special training. We have not got
enough evidence on this yet, but the experience of the next few years
will give us an answer. For the present we cannot too strongly advise
women who are using the method for the second or third time to
perfect their training and increase their chances of success.

Childbirth without pain means effort and knowledge and not
inactivity and ease.

Mme Ameller. Age: 27. Primip. 22 November, 1954. Boy 7 lb 1 oz
When I realized that I was to have a baby, I was somewhat worried.
I knew nothing about medicine. I was a law student, and had heard a
great deal about the terrible sufferings of childbirth.

Fortunately a friend in whom I had great confidence advised me
to try the method, and I went to see Dr V.

I attended the lectures and followed his advice. I did not listen to any more terrible stories about childbirth, and I became full of confidence. A few days before the birth I was completely relaxed and my morale was strong. But the quick respiration was not quite right in spite of my efforts.

The doctor had given the date as between 15 and 20 November. On the night of the 21st – 22nd, I thought the waters had broken. I was not sure. The membranes just leaked. After panicking a little I went back to sleep, and woke at eight feeling well and well rested— unlike my husband. After some preparation and telephone calls I went to the clinic. It was 11.30 a.m., and the doctor happened to be there. He examined me and gave me an injection (aparteine)—the first I had ever had—to make labour start. He advised me to go for a short walk. At about five o'clock I thought I felt the first contractions, and I went back to the clinic and was admitted. Now I was two fingers dilated.

I went to my room and nothing more seemed to happen. I was quite well, much to the surprise of my husband who was still with me and stayed with me all through. At 5.45 a.m. and 6 o'clock I had two more injections (aparteine 5 cg.), and I really felt the first contractions. Then the assistant arrived, and I had to start quick breathing immediately. The contractions became closer, more frequent and prolonged. My breathing was still not quite right, but the assistant helped me to get the right rhythm with unlimited patience and kindness— for which I cannot thank her enough. The contractions became still stronger, and were very frequent but of varying lengths—sometimes one and a half minutes, sometimes only twenty-five to thirty seconds. (This rhythm continued to the end.)

I lost control because of a violent backache and spoilt a contraction —a long one. Then I understood what women who had not tried this method had to suffer. Somebody said, 'You can rub out the pain as you would with a rubber.' I can swear that this is true. The assistant helped me to recover. I managed to ease my back and I felt nothing more till the doctor arrived.

When the baby's head reached the perineum, they said I was breathing more quickly. But I do not remember. It was a reflex. I also had an unfortunate tendency to close my eyes and sleep.

At last came the delivery. It was the time for relaxation, but very short—a few minutes only, ending in an unforgettable moment when I heard the wonderful little creature cry. I pushed twice without effect. At the fifth push I asked if the head were visible, and the doctor brought out the second arm. A few moments later the baby was there on my stomach, and this moment remains engraved on my memory.

I had two clips put in, but this was less painful than an injection, I thought. There was nothing comparable with the atrocious pains borne by so many mothers.

Mme Ameller. Age: 28. Para. 2. 29 January, 1956. Boy 8 lb 13 oz

I had wonderful memories of my first childbirth: I had used the method successfully. My husband, the assistant, the doctor—everyone —played his part at the right moment. I was still more satisfied with it afterwards than at the time of the birth.

But what can I say about the second birth? It went like a flash. Of course, the assistant had told me that everything was quicker for a second baby. For forty-eight hours I had felt the premonitory signs predicted by the doctor, pain in the back, nervousness and especially extreme tiredness and desire to sleep, but I could not believe that my baby would come a good fifteen days in advance.

On Saturday evening, 28 January, at about 10 p.m., I felt two contractions at fifteen minute intervals, but I thought that this was the same as on other nights. However, at the third contraction I told my husband, who wanted to telephone the clinic at once. I would not let him. Then I started having hot and cold sweats and shivers. I thought I had 'flu' and went straight to bed. I noticed then that the mucous plug must have come away, but I had no regular contractions—I had had two at ten minute intervals, then closer together—and I did not want to leave. We had meanwhile told the assistant, and she advised us to wait for regular contractions. Still there was nothing regular. I tried to relax, but I was extremely nervous. At about eleven o'clock the membranes ruptured, and every two minutes, short, and not very strong, contractions started. Now I was really convinced and dressed quickly. My suitcase was ready. I called a friend to look after my son, and we left for the Belvedere. We arrived about 11.30 p.m. This car journey was not at all pleasant. I tried to relax as much as possible, but it was difficult.

I had not yet done any quick breathing.

The midwife's examination showed that I was completely dilated, and the doctor was sent for urgently. He arrived in record time— fifteen minutes—and I found relaxation and quick breathing a great help towards waiting patiently. I did not have to make much effort as the contractions were still short and weak. At this moment my morale was very good. At last I could start pushing. I had not yet got back into training. To my great shame, my strength left me once, but I pushed with all my heart four or five times perhaps. I do not remember. I was thinking so much of concentrating my energies. Then I saw the head of the baby. He gave his first cries, and then the arms came through. He was a boy of 8 lb 11 oz, and my joy was as great as with my first son. It was five minutes past twelve.

The prospect of such happiness should tempt all those who do not believe in the method to try.

By 12.30 p.m. the doctor had gone. I had no tear and no injection. This second success was due mainly to three factors:

1. I had faith in the method, which I had already tried. I had no fear. I listened to the doctor and I believed in what I was doing.

2. I knew that the doctor would not keep me waiting, and this was very important.

3. Finally, I had my husband with me all the time. He was already well-informed, and was perfect at home, in the car and at the clinic. Without him, I should have given way. He helped me to recover my calmness and to bring our son into the world as perfectly as the first.

During my pregnancy, I had two great worries: I was afraid of remaining big and out of shape after two pregnancies. But, having followed the diet prescribed by the doctor, I gained only 17½ lb—the baby's weight was 8 lb 13 oz—and I am slimmer than after the first. This slimness is very important to me. Also a nerve squeezed between two vertebrae had caused violent pains in my back for several months. After a course of massage I had no more pain, but I was afraid it would come back during confinement. The doctor, masseur and assistant all guaranteed to relieve me whatever happened. Little by little, this idea left me, and did not cross my mind at the time. I had no backache at all.

I am really lucky to have had my babies after 1951.

4

Women Difficult to Condition

THIS chapter contains a great variety of reports. They throw light on the most important obstacles to the training of woman. We hope that every future mother who is a special case may find something to think about in them and perhaps solve her own problem. We have divided the cases into two groups:

A. Medical factors.

B. Psychological factors.

A. The medical reasons are easier to explain. So we will begin with them.

When a woman has a disease of the lung, heart, nervous system or anywhere else, she regards herself—and has always been regarded by her family—as not being normal. She herself says: 'I am a sick person.' Until childbirth without pain appeared, pregnancy was thought to make this situation worse. It was considered dangerous, likely to increase existing troubles, and, in certain cases, even a risk to the woman's life. Most abnormalities were regarded as serious and the woman's state of inhibition from the beginning of her pregnancy increased to the maximum. She faced her confinement in the worst possible conditions.

This state of affairs cannot exist with childbirth without pain. The doctor should not neglect any aspect of clinical observation, but he should also try to calm the woman during her pregnancy. She should be looked after more carefully than anyone else. Special examinations should be carried out and repeated to make her confident, and her family circle should be instructed not to frighten her. But also the woman should be shown that she can help herself with training. A pulmonary or cardiac patient learns that if she does not have an anaesthetic during delivery she avoids a risk to herself and her baby. She learns how to economize her efforts and use them intelligently.

She begins to consider herself no longer a special pathological case, but almost normal. Contact with women with similar abnormalities who have already had childbirth without pain will further reassure her.

Many case histories confirm our beliefs.

In C.W.P. everything is possible. We insist on this to doctors who —without proof—deny it.

Of course, in extreme cases pregnancy and confinement can aggravate pre-existing troubles. But the repeated opinions of specialists, before, during and after confinement confirm that C.W.P., far from aggravating pathological conditions, sometimes clears up the subjective troubles related to the diseases.

B. Psychological difficulties are harder to define because many factors are involved. In this field nothing is simple, and there is still much to discover.

One group is particularly difficult to train—women who have had gynaecological treatment for menstrual troubles and especially for 'sterility'. They want a baby very much but consider themselves abnormal and are sure that they cannot accomplish childbirth as perfectly as others. They become anxious during pregnancy and, although during childbirth dilatation may go well, they may fail during delivery. They argue: 'Since I had to go to the doctor for sterility, I am not normal. And so my baby will not be normal either'; and during delivery they go through a period of severe inhibition which makes them lose control.

Equally difficult are the wives of doctors and pediatricians, who are used to hearing about abnormal babies or babies with troubles attributed to childbirth. They fear that their own babies will be malformed, and this anxiety often makes them spoil their delivery. They are afraid of what they are going to see, and so they become completely passive.

Economic and social difficulties are particularly important. The first problem is that of housing. Women in slums or flats fear pregnancy and childbirth because, they say, 'it will make our difficulties still worse.' They feel the same when economic conditions are difficult. There may not be enough money, and a strike may decrease even that; or again the husband may be called up. We have come across this many times in the last few months.

Family difficulties can play an important part. Very often the parents live in a single room with several children. The woman must do her work and carry on without rest or holiday. There is no satisfaction in family life for herself or her husband. Other conflicts appear because the young couple with or without children have to live with 'in-laws', and disagreements arise which upset the couple's own relationship.

A light, pleasant house with plenty of room, enough money and no fear for the future are the best conditions in which a woman can bear a baby. The medical profession should draw the attention of the authorities to this problem, which involves the whole nation. The Government must provide funds for housing and maternal and child welfare. In our opinion, there should be a Ministry of Population, which should aim at improving the physical and moral health of the nation.

Marital difficulties can arise in several ways. A baby may be unwanted by one parent. The husband may see pregnancy as a serious danger to the health or appearance of his wife, and a kind of frustration in the coming of the baby. He may fear that his wife, in devoting herself to the baby, will withold part of her love for him. If training is agreed to, it is possible, with co-operation from wife or husband, to improve such situations and then to change them completely. Successful childbirth will complete the cure.

There are also difficulties in training the unmarried mother who is forsaken by everyone, even, very often, her own family. She fears the birth of her baby, from whom she will very often have to be separated —for the sake of her family or because of financial difficulty. A situation like this must not be allowed to recur. Whatever the circumstances, a mother and child always deserve care. Society must help them instead of rejecting them.

Religious factors have caused serious conflicts in the minds of some women, particularly Catholics. Matters of conscience have arisen which have called for discussion and often much moral courage. In this field, the declaration of the late Pope has clarified the situation. The Catholic woman, now free, will be able—in full harmony with her husband—to educate herself and create life in the moral sense of the term.

Another group of women is particularly difficult to train—those who have lost their first babies, especially if these died during delivery. They want to have a child but are afraid of pregnancy. As soon as they know they are pregnant, they live in daily fear of the confinement. This fear is the greater because they are ignorant of the processes. They read pseudo-medical books or talk about the matter constantly in daily conversation. They are passive during pregnancy, and will be the same during confinement.

They need, more than any other group, to regain confidence in themselves and their capabilities. The doctor has to set their minds at rest, to explain things to them, to make them understand and reassure them. They will need special attention from doctor, midwife and assistant later. They should be isolated as much as possible from the ignorant family circle, and warned against other tattling women. Success will depend on building up a reasoned confidence and turning their passive attitude into something active.

The doctor or midwife should give similar attention to elderly multigravidae, who, as soon as they are pregnant, await their delivery as a terrifying procedure accompanied by fearful accidents.

In all cases, the result would be much better if, at the first visit, the doctor made a list of all the points we have mentioned—physical, psychological, economic, social.

Mme Dietrich. Age: 41. Primip. 25 March, 1955. Girl 6 lb 15 oz. Breech

I was expecting my first baby and I was forty-one years old. It was to be a breech presentation. The child was still in a very high position and a Caesarian was planned if things became complicated.

I regularly attended the lectures on childbirth without pain and was much interested. Each lecture made me discover what childbirth really is. I gradually lost my fears, which had been more or less suggested by my friends on account of my age and the position of the baby. The lectures had explained everything clearly, and I had got an answer to all the questions which worried me. Moreover, I understood that not only my body but my mind and will-power took part in the birth. I knew too that a Caesarian would be only a last resort. I began to trust the method, and I knew that the more I participated the better chance I should have.

On the morning of Friday, 25 March, I felt general tiredness, and I noticed traces of blood. Towards the end of the afternoon I lost the waters. A violent contraction, felt only in the back, followed. I sat down and relaxed for a time. My suitcase was ready, and, though I did not feel like it, I tried to do a few things. I even had enough courage to send my mother home, though she had come to help me in the last moments. At six o'clock new contractions began, still irregular and sharp. I relaxed for a short time. My husband watched me, and I felt he was anxious. I tried not to lose my self-control and automatically the advice and last-minute orders of the assistant came back: 'Keep calm.' Soon, in fact, we both became calm and we had dinner quietly.

It was about seven o'clock. The contractions continued and were more frequent. I told my husband that I would go to the clinic and he wanted to drive me there immediately. . . . But I decided to take my time and get ready as if I was going to the theatre, still following the advice given.

It was 10.30 p.m. when I arrived at the clinic. The midwife examined me. I was only just starting labour, but she decided I should stay. She said delivery would take place the next day, and my husband went back home. I felt lonely and a bit nervous. My baby moved a lot and caused strong contractions in the lumbar region. I did not want to cry out because I had to conserve my strength, and I tried to think of the doctor's last words: 'What a wonderful achievement to bring a baby into the world. . . . It is only you who can make a success of your childbirth.' In the calm of the clinic, I relaxed. It was the beginning of hours of waiting, but I wanted the baby and I was happy.

At 1.30 a.m. I felt my baby coming down gently, and the con-tractions immediately became more regular. I could predict them. There was a slight prickling in the back, and then the wave rose and increased. I started superficial breathing and also long inspirations and expirations. The contractions grew more frequent, still coming from the back. They were at five minute, then four and then three minute intervals. I felt that my body was beyond control, but I was filled with great confidence.

At 6.30 a.m. the midwife examined me and—pleasant surprise!— I heard her say that I was half dilated and labour was normal. She was smiling and so was I because there was now no question of a Caesarian. She telephoned to the doctor and assistant. The assistant arrived almost at once, and the presence of this kind energetic person brought me new comfort and helped me to remain calm. I knew now that all would go well. She massaged me and began the quick respiration with me. She anticipated and guided all my reactions. The contractions were now continuous, and delivery was imminent. I knew exactly what was happening, from what I had been told. Things seemed normal. My assistant decided it was time to go to the labour ward. We went, and I felt her support both physically and morally. My baby came down still further.

The doctor arrived. I was well relaxed, and we noticed this immediately. For a breech, delivery should be quick. He took advantage of a contraction to do an episiotomy (which had been explained to me), and I did not feel it. Now I heard his orders: 'Breathe in, breathe out, stop, push.' Then he said: 'Here are the little buttocks. It's a girl!' I gave a second push. This time I felt my baby coming out of my body —an unforgettable experience.

The doctor put my little Claire on my stomach (eight o'clock). What joy when I touched my baby for the first time—really alive and giving her first cry.

Words cannot express what I felt then for the doctor and his assistants. It was more than gratitude.

Mme Planadevall. Age: 33. Primip. 9 November, 1954. Boy 8 lb 10 oz

Before describing my confinement, I should mention my state of mind when pregnancy started. A complete change took place between the beginning of pregnancy and childbirth, a change which greatly surprised my family and friends.

I am abnormally afraid of pain, not only in myself but in another human being or animal. Even at the cinema I cannot stand the sight of a surgical operation or even injection, and accidents, blood or wounds are worse. So I contemplated childbirth with terror, having heard all the stories of its torture from other women. I feared motherhood much more than a surgical operation—which at least is carried out under complete anaesthesia. I had come to feel repulsion for children who had brought torment to their mothers, and, of course, I did not want any. It was a catastrophe for me when I found I was pregnant. I was completely desperate. I thought of suicide. I felt like an animal caught in a trap from which it cannot escape.

However, things being as they were, I had to choose a clinic. I had read articles on childbirth without pain and had heard a broadcast on one of these confinements. The method seemed intelligent and logical. It appealed to me greatly. One thing made me hesitate. I had no confidence in myself. Though the method was excellent for women of normal sensibilities, could it be used for me whose state of mind was so deplorable?

Yet by traditional methods, I was sure to suffer. The new method left me with a hope, a chance. If it failed, it could not be worse than other systems.

So I made up my mind. But I did not immediately acquire confidence. I had moments of terrible depression, and many fits of crying. Fear was always in my mind like a shadow. My pregnancy progressed, and the time for training came at last. I started this with the same anxieties, wondering if I could summon up enough strength to control my fear, and do what was necessary. I had many doubts. My assistant can vouch for this. But I worked hard, did what I was told and followed the doctor's lectures with the greatest interest.

Just when I was going to see the film I had another terrible fit of depression—the last. It was about a month before term, and suddenly the confidence I had gained with so much difficulty left me. I was advised not to see the film, but something made me go. I took the risk; either this would finish me or would do me a lot of good.

It did me a lot of good. I, who cannot stand seeing an injection, easily stood the sight of this childbirth because it was obvious that the woman did not suffer.

From that moment, everything changed for me. My terror disappeared. For the last fifteen days of my pregnancy I was in excellent spirits. And then came the great day. It was 9 November. At 4.30 a.m. I woke up and could not go back to sleep. I was calmly thinking of my future childbirth at 5.30 a.m. when I felt the first contractions. They were completely painless. I waited more than an hour still lying down, so that I could study them. Their irregularity (ten, five or fifteen minutes) surprised me. But I got up to be ready whatever happened, and washed and dressed with a calmness which astonished me. Then my husband took me to the nursing home. I was examined at ten o'clock. I was not dilated at all, and I was sent back home. I was having no more contractions.

The only pains I had were caused by my clumsiness when I took the prescribed enema. I had a few intestinal pains because I injected some air. But these passed very quickly, and I went on knitting. Then I had a good lunch, and a friend came in the afternoon. There were no other warning signs except that in the middle of the afternoon the mucous plug came away. At about 5.30 p.m. the contractions returned more strongly. I lay down on my bed and knitted quietly. During the contraction I did the quick breathing which stopped any unpleasant feeling. I failed once or twice to synchronize the contraction and the breathing, and I noticed that I then had pain. Between the contractions I relaxed well and I breathed deeply.

I went to the nursing home with my husband. In the taxi I put my feet on the folding seat and remained still, completely relaxed and calm—much to my surprise.

I reached the nursing home at 8.25 p.m. I was examined and

innocently asked the midwife if labour had started. To my great surprise, she said that I was between one-half and three-quarters dilated, and it was time to call the doctor and assistant.

While I was waiting for them, the membranes were ruptured and the contractions immediately became stronger. I continued quick respiration with deep breathing in between. I was still calm. The doctor and assistant arrived shortly after, and delivery started.

I began to push according to instructions. I had to make great efforts, because a few small difficulties arose. The back of the baby was to the right, the head very big and the ligament on the right of the pelvis very hard. Also I felt no urge to push.

Anyhow I did my best, according to what I had been taught, though at the beginning I made a few mistakes in breathing. The doctor had to help me with forceps. But there again I felt no pain. The only unpleasant thing was to have to push, to make this great muscular effort and to stand the resulting heat. At 9.15 p.m. the baby was born, one and a half hours after I had arrived at the nursing home. I had hardly felt the delivery, which I had previously imagined would be butchery. I just felt the tissues stretched painlessly. I remained fully aware until the end and careful to do all that was necessary.

Although the forceps were used, I had no tear. I was not damaged at all. I was able to give birth without pain, and I have remarkable memories of this event.

Psychologically, this absence of suffering had very important consequences. I, who thought of the arrival of a baby as a calamity, who had no maternal instinct—because, I realize now, I was afraid of suffering—and who even thought that I could not become fond of the baby, am very happy to have him. Besides, I feel freed from an obsession. I no longer fear another childbirth.

My husband's support greatly assisted me. He, too, believed in the value of the method, and he helped me do the exercises. During confinement he remained quite calm, and this strengthened my own determination.

From the bottom of my heart I thank the doctor and my assistant, Mme D., whose advice was a great help. I know that if I had given birth by another method I should have been completely panic-stricken and incapable of controlling my fear.

Mme Le Flem. Age: 27. Para. 2 (first dead). 3 February, 1954. Boy 7 lb 2 oz
On 3 February I gave birth without pain; yes, without pain. But

words are powerless to express all that I have just experienced! I have had a wonderful adventure with the training for this childbirth, and now that Alan is born I feel that I have passed a difficult exam. I have won a race, which I thought at first I could not undertake. It is a bit like being uncertain about an athlete, who ends up as champion.

Only seventeen months ago, Yves was born, our first child. We lost him when he was four days old. He was born with an umbilical hernia, and an operation was tried but failed. This was a shock, and I was still affected by the loss when I became pregnant again. I had to be deconditioned from my fears and anxieties about the health of our second baby, and also from all the terrible memories of my first childbirth. I had forty-eight hours alone in a room at the nursing home with a labour which made no progress. Finally, after induction of dilatation, I had forceps, episiotomy, anaesthetics. After all this pain—to lose my baby! It was a nightmare for many months. I was tormented by it. In any case I have a nervous temperament!

Then one of my cousins, who had just very successfully experienced childbirth without pain, managed to convince me. At the beginning of my second pregnancy I went to see the doctor. I must have made a bad impression at this first visit. I told him, with tears, about my first childbirth and the loss of our little Yves, whom we had wanted so much. I felt that he had doubts about me, though I know now that he has confidence in us all. But I was a bad subject from the start.

Today I cry 'Victory', like thousands of happy mothers. I have won in spite of my hypersensitive mentality. The method has been proved once more. With my husband, I attended the doctor's lectures and the training at the assistant's. Each time I came away enriched and transformed, discovering more and more of the marvels of pregnancy and childbirth. I grew more confident in myself, full of new strength and hope which would be completely realized at the birth of our second baby.

This birth was like a dream coming true. I was so well prepared that I wanted intensely to experience it, to have my turn. Term approached, and I was not the least bit afraid or doubtful. I understood exactly what was going to happen, and I wanted to follow consciously the whole course of labour, the whole phase of dilatation—adapting myself as we had learned—and then delivery, the most wonderful stage. This time I wanted to make my baby come into the world!

And everything went well, as the doctor had said it would. This is the wonderful thing about the training. Everything the doctor or assistant says is true.

The doctor told us that there was a difficult moment— between three-quarters and full dilatation, when the contractions change and when one feels the first need to push! It is true. This desire to push is very strong and one must know how to adapt to it in a new way by quick breathing. At that time, the help of the assistant and my husband was just what I wanted. I also knew that I was going to the labour ward where I should find the doctor!

Childbirth was very quick.

From the Monday I had felt some contractions, but they were irregular. On Tuesday I had lumbar pains, and I was sorry to be sleeping so badly, knowing that term was near. On Wednesday night the lumbar pains took up a regular rhythm, and we decided to go to the clinic. It was 10 p.m. when we arrived. The midwife examined me. (Her examination was very gentle and there was a great difference from my arrival at the other clinic for my first confinement.) She said that labour had only just started and birth would take place the next day. I therefore stayed at the clinic—mainly so that I could sleep.

After an injection of coramine-spasmaverine, I went to sleep with no worries, but was woken up several times by the lumbar pains. During the night I had another injection of spasmaverine, and when the assistant arrived about 10 o'clock she found me still dozing! I was happy that time had passed so quietly because some of the labour was accomplished, and when I really woke up I was two fingers dilated.

Straight away Mme D. and I did quick superficial breathing. The presence of the assistant at your side plays a very big part towards the success of childbirth without pain. I felt guided and protected by her. She gave me strength, being very energetic and at the same time very gentle. Two or three times I showed signs of impatience, wanting to push, though it was still not time, and I received two little slaps from her which did me a lot of good!

I felt however that she was not too dissatisfied with me. I had given her a few worries during my training. At first I had done badly the movements for delivering, and I found muscular relaxation very difficult. My success later on I owe first to the assistant but also very much to my husband, who supervised me and made me repeat the exercises every night.

The assistant helped me not to give way. The contractions immediately became quite strong, and then light massage on my stomach did me a lot of good. I managed to time my breathing and do some deep breathing as well. I did this because I had learned that, if the respiration is not started at the beginning of the contraction, this can become painful and create a serious conditioned reflex. So, between contractions, I tried to recover by relaxing as much as possible. Also Mme D. gave me something to drink and cooled me with a damp sponge. I was very hot and my mouth was completely dry.

At 5 a.m. the membranes were ruptured quite painlessly. At the same time I had an injection of dolosal because of the rigidity of my cervix. My husband arrived about 11 a.m. While the assistant kept an eye on me, he helped me to adapt my breathing and timed the length and frequency of the contractions. From then on these became stronger and stronger and closer together. They were only two minutes apart and they lasted one and a quarter minutes and some nearly one and a half minutes. Labour progressed rapidly. I was half and then three quarters dilated. I have already said I found the transition from three quarters to complete dilatation difficult, but then rapid respiration helped me to carry on. It is incredible how much I wanted to go to the labour ward! During the lectures the doctor had made me impatient to experience the actual birth of my baby. He knew how to describe it to us as so beautiful, rich in meaning and full of emotion! There too, during delivery, complete adaptation is necessary and I understand now why, without this adaptation, delivery can be long and very difficult.

How happy I was to leave for the labour ward. I was a bit like the child who goes on Christmas morning to the fireplace, knowing that something wonderful and new is waiting. But what exactly? What surprise will he find? I felt like that.

And I was not robbed of my joy or surprise. I experienced an exciting delivery. Active, careful but calm, relaxed when necessary, I felt my baby coming down. In three pushes, I gave birth to him. I was dissatisfied because I spoilt one, going on breathing when I should have stopped, but I pulled myself together very quickly.

One thing: I am sorry I did not ask for an injection of caffeine to stimulate me more. I wanted to be still more alert and attentive during delivery.

What is extraordinary in this phase is our conditioning to the words of the doctor! The words: 'Breathe in. . . . Breathe out. . . .

Stop. . . . Push. . . .' really inspired me. Our ability to obey the words, and especially the doctor's order—'Again. . . . Again. . . . Again . . .'— while we push, is surprising!

The head reached the perineum, and the doctor announced, as he had said he would, 'The hair. . . . The head. . . . The forehead, the eyes, the whole head, the first shoulder. . . .' I had clearly before my eyes the pictures in the film which I have seen eight days before. I needed to digest this film, having been greatly struck by the pictures. Now I realize that it plays a basic part in the training, more especially as we see it at the end of the course when we are ready. It is a synthesis and a revision.

It is essential to relax completely when the doctor says: 'Don't push any more,' and I managed to relax so that I felt nothing when my perenium tore again. (It was scarred.) I repeat I felt nothing, and I had no pain at any time.

At 1.25 p.m. Alan was born. They showed him to me. He was put on my stomach, but before that I had felt his little arm on me. Then, like so many mothers, I bent forward to see him and take him.

How happy I was when my baby first cried, so happy that I kissed Mme D., the assistant. The doctor was busy with the cord, then the placenta, and Alan had his first wash. I was not at all tired! It was done. I had managed it. The doctor, my husband and the assistant had put their confidence in me, and I had not disappointed them. But the next time. . . . I think about it already. Isn't it surprising? I want to do better still.

My husband, wearing a white coat, was at my side in the labour ward, I needed him. His eyes were shining with tears when Alan was born. He, too, must have tasted this unique joy. He helped me to train and made me believe in success. We have conquered it, both of us together, this childbirth without pain, and from this birth we emerge enriched. We have lived unforgettable moments that will be good to remember. The doctor had told us this too. 'The husband must take part in and be present at the childbirth.'

A very important point. At the beginning of the morning, when dilatation had scarcely started, I was fortunate in being visited by the doctor, quite unexpectedly! It was a stimulus, for he told me rather severely: 'You understand, don't you? You are not to think about your first confinement.' And in fact I gave no thought to it at any time. I was completely deconditioned and, knowing that my baby was going to be born, I did not even think that he might be deformed like the first baby. The doctor knew how to give me confidence, to condition me to expect a healthy and beautiful baby, I shall never forget the tone of his voice when he said: 'A normal boy, quite normal.' This too is a victory. A victory I owe to the method.

My impressions? To have had childbirth without pain has removed the age-long idea of the sufferings of childbirth. For many centuries these pains were accepted as part of the female condition. Now these prejudices are uprooted from my mind and my husband's, and we shall tell everybody about it. Instead of submitting to this pain, we know how to overcome it by training and overcome it naturally— quite conscious, quite free. It is our victory; this childbirth belongs to us women. We must acquire it, but it is a gift to the baby, a gift to the husband. I understood this from my own husband's look which showed how proud he was of me.

Childbirth without pain beautifies motherhood, because a birth in these conditions is a wonderful thing! No more contorted, unapproachable women, wincing, writhing and screaming on their beds. The future mother is dignified, calm, relaxed, smiling, even during her efforts. She has a clear look, thinking not of her own suffering, but of the baby, whom she is going to see coming into the world, and of those who are around her.

Nobody can tell me that with this method one might love the baby less! It is impossible! I am drunk with happiness when I gaze at our little Alan. I am entranced by him. I have a gentle peace deep down in me, as after a job well done. This is because one must work to succeed. Will-power, enthusiasm, perseverance and confidence are needed during the training and, when the time comes, a lot of self-control and concentration.

Although I seem guilty of pride, I can consider my childbirth without pain as a victory over myself—who am so worried, so impressionable! Already I feel stronger. It is a new 'me' which I have discovered. Every woman who uses childbirth without pain must find new possibilities in herself which perhaps she had no idea of!

Birth with this method is truly an incomparable blossoming out.

Note: As a Catholic, I had scruples right at the beginning about training myself by this method. Did not the terrible words: 'You will have children in pain' imply an obligation? Was I not going to betray my faith?

I asked my confessor for advice. He was definite, and said: 'Don't worry. You're going to give birth without pain. That means naturally, and it doesn't exclude all the moral difficulties, tiredness and worries which bringing up a child means. This, too, is meant by Christ's prophecy, 'You will have children in pain.' And he added, because he knew of the method, 'You will have your baby joyfully, and all real joy brings you to God and glorifies Him.'

Not long ago the whole Church adopted this position on childbirth without pain—it had to—and all Catholics are happy because of it.

Mme Jouhaud. Age: 30. Para. 3. 18 April, 1955. Girl 6 lb 11 oz

On 18 April, at three in the morning, I brought into the world, in the full sense of the words, my third daughter. My first two children are five and four years old. In my previous confinements I spent about two hours screaming like a wild beast; then I had an anaesthetic. When I came round, they gave me a baby bound up in its nappy, washed and dressed. I was, of course, very happy to hold it in my arms, but I contemplated it with the hidden disappointment of not having participated in its birth and with an indefinable feeling of emptiness, due to the gap in time.

When childbirth without pain made its appearance in France and articles started to appear in the newspapers, my interest was immediately awakened, and I devoured the issue of *Regards* devoted to the subject. Since then I have read with pleasure and increasing interest all the information that came from Dr. Lamaze's clinic or from his colleagues—which I picked up here and there.

In August, 1954, I was pregnant. I immediately contacted a friend who had experienced childbirth without pain two years earlier, and she recommended me to the doctor. Before the first visit, I was already convinced of the value of the method, and after a few minutes' conversation I was full of confidence.

I have had poliomyelitis, and I still show the effects of the attack I had in 1929 when I was five years old—almost complete paralysis of the right leg, severe muscle and bone wasting which have meant wearing an iron. In addition, the pelvis was affected and shows considerable asymmetry. The doctor did not conceal that I might come up against some difficulties during my confinement (the weight of the baby even to a few ounces more or less being important) but it would not in any way prevent me from delivering my baby properly.

The first three months of my pregnancy were a bit unpleasant, with rather frequent nausea, but later it went on very well. The doctor's lectures and the practical training with Mlle H. enthralled me. I worked very conscientiously and trained myself regularly every day.

During the night of 13–14 April I began to lose the waters and to have a few contractions, but they were completely irregular. In the morning my husband took me to the nursing home where they found no dilatation at all. The membranes were only leaking. On the doctor's advice, I stayed nearby and had a very pleasant day—lunch at a restaurant, then the cinema in the afternoon with my husband. I had some contractions which seemed to become regular for a time; then they disappeared. They were not very strong, and I had no difficulty in controlling them. What worried me most was that, at the same time, I felt severe pains in the small of the back for which nothing can be done. They reminded me very unpleasantly of my previous confinements.

I returned to the nursing home about six o'clock and had an injection to speed up labour. I went out again with my husband, and came back about 8.20 p.m. I had had some stronger contractions, nearly regular, but again they became less frequent. Examination showed that there was no change, but, for safety, I spent the night at the nursing home. The next morning the contractions had completely stopped, and my husband came to fetch me. The days of the 15th and 16th passed. I went on losing a little, and at times I had very bad pain in the back. On Sunday the 17th I had quite a lot to do in the house—bathing my daughter, cleaning, cooking, etc.—whereas the two previous days I had sat down almost all the time.

'Needs must'; and after all, I thought, perhaps rushing about like this would hurry things up. During the afternoon I had to stop what I was doing several times to control a contraction.

As they were not at all regular, it did not occur to me to go to the nursing home. At 5.30 p.m. I accompanied my husband to the town hall to vote, and scarcely had we returned when the contractions came on regularly. I got dinner ready quickly, and while we were eating they came every five minutes. It was eight o'clock. I put my daughter to bed and gave myself an enema, and we left a little after nine o'clock. We had telephoned Mlle H., whom we picked up at her home. Throughout the journey the contractions occurred every five minutes. I did quick respiration, with perfect control and had no uterine pain. If it were not for that wretched backache!

After arriving at the nursing home I went to bed, and Mlle H. and my husband sat near me. I was perfectly calm and relaxed. While talking I let two contractions take hold, but I did not let it happen again!

The pain in the back was continual and became stronger with each contraction. It was through this that I detected the contractions, because they were not very typical, the uterus staying hard and contracted and not relaxing between them. Mlle H. added to the relief obtained from quick breathing by lightly massaging my lower abdomen.

At two o'clock the contractions were coming about every three minutes. I was beginning to feel tired, and I was overwhelmed by the bone pains. I made huge efforts to control myself and not to become tense. My two watchers did not relax their attention, and I clung to their care and their voices. After 2.30 a.m. I was taken to the labour ward. The face of Doctor R., so nice and so calm—although he had just finished his second delivery—stimulated me further, but not for long.

When the time of delivery came, after I had pushed twice, the doctor said: 'You won't be able to push him out. The head is not at all flexed. I have to turn it. After that everything will be all right.' During the rotation, I gave way for a few minutes. I got tense, and as a result had a very painful cramp in one leg and I screamed. Only once, but I screamed. Immediately I heard the doctor's voice, firm, calm, kind. 'There, it's done. It's your turn now. Breathe in, breathe out, breathe in, stop, push.' I was reconditioned. I had pulled myself together, and in three or four pushes the head appeared. 'Another push for the shoulder,' and I felt a little warm arm on my thigh. I raised myself and saw my baby. The doctor finished the delivery and put her on my stomach: 'Here is your daughter.' I knew it was an extraordinary moment, but words are powerless to express one's feelings.

About ten minutes later the placenta was delivered very easily, and they took me back to my room. My husband departed. He had not left me for a minute, and in the difficult moments his presence had been particularly precious. His complete calm was one of the factors which helped me to pull myself together quickly.

Before going to sleep, I relived the hours which had just passed and of course I was upset at having lost control for a moment. Still, I was overcome with the joy of having given birth to my baby myself.

The day after, when I saw Dr. V. and Dr. R., both assured me that the bad time was caused by the shape of my pelvis and that I managed very well. They were both wonderfully kind, but it seems to me that I could have done better. My daughter weighed 6 lb 11 oz—the others were 5 lb 10 oz and 6 lb 5 oz—and it is very likely, as Dr. V. said, that she was a little bit too big for my pelvis.

So I went through the test of childbirth without pain. Brilliantly?

No. Successfully? Yes. And if I should go through it once more in the future, my strongest wish will be to pass with distinction. There is one thing I want to add. I was in a room with two beds, and the day after a woman came in, a primip. forty-two years old, whose contractions were coming about every quarter of an hour. She was beginning to find them very hard to bear, and I briefly explained to her how she should relax and breathe. It was then five o'clock in the morning. Until ten o'clock—the contractions were coming then at less than five-minute intervals and lasted a very long time—she managed to control herself very well for someone who had not been trained. I helped her as best as I could, talking to her and encouraging her and breathing in time with her. Finally, she controlled herself no longer, and she went to the labour ward where she was anaesthetized for the birth of her daughter. She is very grateful to me for having helped her to hold out for five hours, and if she has other children she will train herself for childbirth without pain.

Note from the father:
I wish to add my evidence to that of my wife. I think it important for the success of childbirth without pain that the husband should not be absent, or simply a spectator, more or less embarrassed and in the way. In my wife's two previous confinements I literally ran away from the nursing home when she started to scream worse than an animal. This time I attended the whole training with her, the doctor's lectures and the midwife's practical classes. I tried to help her to do her exercises each day, and I discussed magazine articles and books that we read on psychoprophylactic childbirth.

What most surprised me in retrospect was how calm we were when we went to the nursing home on the day. We had to drive about thirty miles in the suburbs of Paris, and I have seldom driven so quickly and with so much self-control. The contractions were coming every five minutes, and we knew that things happened quickly in multiparous women.

Actually my wife took six hours. I stayed with her all the time, helping her to control her contractions and relax when the midwife had to leave. There were four deliveries that night. And when the doctor used forceps to turn the baby's head, I was of some use because I helped him to recondition my wife who had become tense and was screaming. I do not know if I could have done it if I had not attended the training. Untrained, I should perhaps have reacted badly and been a cause of failure, as happens sometimes with C.W.P. in the country when the family is against it.

I do not know if we shall have any more children. In any case, Sylvie's birth will be the most moving memory of my life. It is the first birth of one of my children where I was happy and in complete harmony with my wife.

Mme Youenou. Age: 25. Para. 2 (first dead). 7 April, 1954. Boy 7 lb 15 oz

I started my second pregnancy with the memory of my first confinement. It was carried out traditionally with injections, anaesthetics and forceps. The baby was born with two marks on its temples and died three hours later. After a test, an abnormality of the blood was found. My husband was Rhesus positive and I was Rhesus negative, which made us very worried about another pregnancy, though we wanted a child very much. My husband was advised on the matter by a colleague who was enthusiastic about his wife's confinement. Dr. — had carried it out without pain or anaesthetic, and my husband decided to consult this doctor. My first visit to him reassured me, although I am naturally a very anxious person. During the following months I had regular blood tests at St. Antoine's Hospital, and paid monthly visits to the doctor. These gave me confidence. At the sixth month of my pregnancy the classes with the assistant began—breathing exercises for each phase of confinement, physical exercises to loosen the muscles, and pushing for delivery. The exercises had to be repeated every night. I did not seem very apt in muscular relaxation and this gap in my training worried me. Quick and deep respiration made progress.

On the evening of 6 April, after my last visit to the doctor, I felt the first contraction, showing that childbirth was beginning. I told my husband and we waited, carrying on as usual. We slept until two in the morning. The contractions were a bit closer together, but I felt no pain and I was completely relaxed. What had worried me so much took place without any effort. I dozed until morning and began breathing deeply between contractions; then I thought it was time to go to the clinic.

About eleven o'clock, in the labour ward, the midwife found that dilatation had reached three fingers. The contractions followed each other regularly and without pain. The breathing helped me all the time. Then the assistant and doctor arrived. After the membranes were ruptured, the contractions came more frequently, and the time arrived to start quick respiration. I was helped by the assistant, who told me what to do and gave me the rhythm as the contractions increased. The doctor kept an eye on the progress of labour. When he told me, 'In fifteen minutes the baby will be here,' I did not believe him because I felt so well.

Soon after, I had an urgent desire to push, and the doctor warned me 'Not yet.' Quick breathing still helped me, but the desire to push increased. 'Breathe in, stop, push.' I did it twice very hard. 'Quick breathing.' I felt the baby slide down. Then, 'Look at your baby.' My son, still quite blue, was on my stomach. The doctor tied the cord, and a midwife took the baby to wash and weigh him: 7 lb 15 oz. He was a big boy. The perineum, which had been badly damaged during my first confinement, had now been only slightly torn. One stitch was enough.

I am still amazed by the speed of it all and the atmosphere of confidence in the labour ward. I was not afraid at all. I knew exactly what the doctor and his assistants were doing; a revision lecture had prepared me for it. And now that I know, I shall give birth only in this way.

A note from the husband:

The night of 6 April, when she came back from seeing the doctor, Jacqueline felt the first slight contractions indicating childbirth. We did nothing special. She slept until two in the morning, and then the contractions became more obvious and regular. They continued like this and she slept lightly. Her morale was as good as possible. During her pregnancy they had been determined to reduce my wife's main emotional reaction—the anxiety engendered by the failure of her first confinement (eighteen painful hours, only to lose her son) and by her vague obsessions about serological factors. The doctor's devotion to the future mother was in the best Hippocratic tradition.

When we arrived at the nursing home at about eleven o'clock, Jacqueline was three fingers dilated. She breathed deeply during each contraction. In between, I talked without asking her questions. She was very calm, mentally and physically, in spite of her half-sleepless night. I felt she was as confident as a child who is sure he knows his lessons. She applied her training—deep normal oxygenation, like an athlete before exertion, and relaxation. (I was a bit anxious on this score.) The midwife came regularly to see the results. The cervix dilated; the doctor came to rupture the membrane, which made the contractions stronger and more frequent.

Jacqueline practised breathing quickly. Mme C., the assistant, was there, and now this mysterious phenomenon of transference took place. Jacqueline confidently put herself in the hands of the assistant, who took control of the labour. To avoid breathlessness, she used the oxygen mask. 'Contraction is starting. Breathe normally. Breathe in. Breathe out. . . .' While the assistant directed the rhythm and guided Jacqueline by breathing quickly herself, her hand worked and massaged my wife's perineum. This helped a lot, she told me later.

At about 11.50 a.m. the contractions were very strong. I was very happy that Jacqueline held on; there was no panic as the contraction arrived. Physiologically the need for oxygen was satisfied, and I suppose that—with the quick breathing—the sensation of pain was delayed. Because of this, I waited for her to cry out. 'The baby is pressing on the rectum,' the assistant said. Mme C.'s calmness and authority stopped my wife from letting herself push as she would have liked.

It was midday. The doctor was at the foot of the table. 'It hurts,' said Jacqueline. 'Breathe in, stop, push . . .' ordered the assistant. Twice: the baby suddenly came out. Jacqueline was the only one who did not see him.

'Look at your baby,' said Mme C., and she put him on her stomach, connected by the umbilical cord, the size of which surprised me. She smiled at her son, strong in her mother's joy. The delivery of the placenta was easily accomplished. Our team broke up; everyone left. Jacqueline rested.

Though I am easily impressionable, I wanted to be present throughout the confinement. Nothing frightening happened—nothing but an act, naturally carried out, among medical attendants, competent, kind and humane.

5

Medical and Auxiliary Medical Professions

I T may seem surprising to devote a section to reports on the childbirth of women doctors, doctors' wives, midwives and women in
auxiliary medical professions. We do this for two main reasons:

1. These reports have a different significance from those of other
women. They have more authority as assertions of the method's value.

2. This group of women is difficult to train. All have medical
knowledge and often knowledge of obstetrics. They remember their
courses in hospitals where childbirth without pain was not used. It
seems impossible, almost unimaginable, to them. They must make a
very great effort to forget what they know on the subject. A woman
who submits herself to instruction and training and forgets her profession can succeed like any other woman. But if she does not wish to
study the method as an ordinary pupil, she risks failure.

Childbirth without pain is not reserved for specific types of women.
The intellectural as well as the labourer's wife can benefit from it,
provided that she works with the same application.

Women help one another during the training. They take an interest
in each other and try especially to assist those with the greatest difficulties. This collaboration is always valuable.

Finally, how persuasive a woman doctor can be, when she has had
the experience. When she talks to other women or her colleagues,
she knows better than anyone else how to explain and convince.

Report of Dr. B., a woman doctor.
I got into touch with the team of childbirth without pain for one of
my patients. She was a young neurotic woman, with agarophobia,
who had said many times since the beginning of her marriage that she
did not want to have children because she was too much afraid of the
pains of childbirth. Childbirth might plunge her into an irreversible

psychosis, or, on the other hand, draw her out of her state of apathy, passiveness and indifference to life. I counted mainly on the psychological training of the constant presence of an assistant or doctor during confinement.

The psychological training was not perfect. As it happened, my patient attended group classes given by the assistant, and there was not the intimacy that I should have liked for her. She was especially frightened by the physical effort which she would have to make and which was insisted upon; she had not the energy at that time to lift a saucepan full of water. I had warned the assistant and asked her to be there from the beginning of labour because I feared a disaster.

I was present throughout her confinement. Labour was very quick for a primipara—six hours. Throughout, though she was usually weak, anxious and plaintive about the smallest thing, my patient remained perfectly calm and relaxed. She told me that the contractions were hardly painful with the quick breathing. She only wanted to know if 'the pain would not become worse'.

She was then almost completely dilated. During delivery, I was struck by a change in her behaviour. She was pushing strongly and energetically, exactly following the doctor's instructions.

The only false note was her repulsion when she saw the baby. I think that this was one of the consequences of psychological training in a group which had not conditioned her enough.

This result seemed sensational to me, and the more so as the assistant was prevented by unforeseen circumstances from attending. My patient was guided at the start by her husband and myself and then by the doctor.

I came out of the labour ward quite bowled over. We heard no cries or groans. I was all the more amazed because I remembered my own confinement.

It had taken place fifteen months previously, in May 1953. I had not been anxious. I wanted this baby. The pregnancy had been normal. The presentation was good, and the doctor had promised me a good anaesthetic with nitrous oxide as soon as I was three fingers dilated.

Labour was very long (twenty-four hours). It started with little, not very painful, contractions for eight to nine hours; then the contractions became more frequent and stronger.

I was then two fingers dilated. I was calm between contractions but became very restless during the pains which radiated strongly in the lumbar region. I was then given my first injection of spasmalgine.

The pains became a little less intense and further apart. Another injection of spasmalgine was given four hours later. I was then nearly three fingers dilated, and it was 2 a.m.

I was taken to the labour ward, and the anaesthetist began to give me nitrous oxide during the contractions. At the first pain, all went well. I was relieved, only vaguely conscious of an unpleasant abdominal tension. Then the anaesthetic stopped working. I began to get restless, especially because I was afraid of the bad effect of a prolonged anaesthetic on the baby. I lost all control of myself, I, who was proud of my powers of resistance. I began to scream and struggle so much that my husband had to hold me. My state was due, I think, to several causes. The nitrous oxide, in acting partly but not enough on the cortex, had freed the subcortical centres; and to the intense pain was added anxiety because the anaesthetic was not working and I was alone with my husband. The midwife was busy with another delivery.

At 5 a.m. the midwife rang up the doctor to tell him that labour was not progressing much, and that I was very restless. Then the membranes ruptured. The doctor was told, and he considered that labour would progress more rapidly.

For two hours more I fought under the mask, screaming continuously. My husband could not stand it, and urged the midwife to telephone the doctor. At about seven o'clock I felt that the pains were changing, and I recognized the delivery pains. I wanted to push, but the midwife was busy elsewhere and the anaesthetist asked me to wait and tried to give more anaesthetic—without effect. This scene of Grand Guignol—myself screaming, struggling and pushing in a completely uncontrolled way, my husband holding me, the anaesthetist not knowing what to do—lasted fifty minutes. Then, after two telephone calls, the doctor at last arrived. I was put deeply asleep, and when I woke up my first thought was to find out if the baby had cried immediately and whether he was a mongol. I remained prostrated the whole day, exhausted not as much by the labour as by the restlessness and anxiety which had taken hold of me throughout the night.

I have described my confinement with all these details to show how my husband and I, who wanted a second baby quickly, were hesitating at the prospect of a similar ordeal. I had read some articles on childbirth without pain and the Pavlovian method, but I had no personal ideas on this subject. The guided confinement under spinal anaesthesia seemed to me very interesting for the mother but dangerous for the baby.

I was five months pregnant when I was present at the confinement of my patient. I made up my mind.

I insisted on following the whole training scrupulously, both with the assistant and doctor. I did not learn anything new because I had read all that had been written on childbirth without pain, and I knew Pavlovian physiology, but the training kept me in a cheerful state of mind. The confinement ceased to seem a nightmare and appeared an exciting experience in which I could take an active part. Labour would be real work to which I was growing accustomed. There would be different phases, and I was taught my part for each.

Labour began on 21 July at 5.45 a.m. with a vague feeling of pain in the pelvis. At 6 o'clock came a new tightness, a really painful contraction which lasted a few seconds. At 6.15 a.m. there was another contraction. As I was expecting it, I did the deep respiration with light massage of the lower abdomen. I thought that this contraction was less painful than the previous one. From now on the contractions followed more closely every ten and then five minutes. The deep breathing was no longer any help, so I did the quick breathing, but the conditions were bad because I had got up to take a shower and dress. At seven o'clock we left home. In the few yards to the car I had a very long and painful contraction that quick respiration, as I was standing up, did not control. I was able to judge in this way the help which breathing brought me in the car where I had had three contractions and where, in spite of the jolts, they were easily bearable. At the clinic, where we arrived at 7.15, the contractions became still more frequent. The midwife quickly examined me and found me three fingers dilated. At once she telephoned to the doctor to come. I did the quick respiration almost without stopping because the contractions were still more frequent and strong. In this stage I went through a few very unpleasant minutes. I had a strong desire to push, and, in spite of the exhortations of my assistant who was there for another delivery, I got restless.

Conditions were bad, for I was on a divan, the four labour wards being occupied. Labour took place very quickly, so that I did not have time to adapt myself to the rhythm of the contractions. Finally, still because of the speed of labour, I had reached complete dilatation before the doctor arrived. He came at 7.50 a.m., and at last I could push. In four pushes the head was at the vulva. These pushes were completely painless. I felt the head moving and stretching the perineum, but I had no pain at all. Then the doctor said: 'Relax now,' and I heard him describe the forehead emerging, the nose, the chin and finally the whole head.

Then came one of the arms. I smiled because, forgetting that I was a doctor and had seen new-born babies, the doctor said: 'And remember that he is blue.' It was then that I saw the baby and heard his first cry. The placenta also came extremely easily. At 8.20 a.m. it was all over —labour and delivery of the placenta. I had a cup of tea and put on some lipstick. I was still amazed at the ease and joy with which I had brought my baby into the world. I telephoned my parents an hour later to tell them of the birth of their grandson.

These two confinements, so different, if only because of their atmosphere, will no doubt raise critical comment.

Certainly it was a second confinement and a very quick labour. However, it is said in all the obstetrics text-books that uterine contraction is characterized by pain. Now, although I cannot say that the contractions were completely painless, they were perfectly bearable, and I was not restless and did not groan at a stage where, physiologically, the contraction was at its peak. The only bad moment was when I wanted to push but could not. This period would have been more bearable if I had been more comfortable with the doctor beside me.

The speed of the labour is an interesting thing to note. It occurred with my patient as well, and, in the many case histories I have read, I have been struck with it—even in primiparous women. Is this the result of the breathing and relaxation, or of the training in the days preceding confinement?

Whatever it is, I consider that this method should be enforced in all maternity clinics. In view of the results, it seems unthinkable that lack of money or personnel can be given as an excuse or that anybody can pretend that 'a good anaesthetic or spinal costs less and works just as well'. Apart from the joy the mother feels at seeing her baby come into the world, the new method is harmless, whereas anaesthesia may not be.

The 'primum non nocere' claimed today for proprietary preparations should not become just a laboratory motto, but must remain the first principle of the doctor's practice.

Mme Dutilleul, ex-midwife. Age: 29. Primip. 5 February, 1954. Boy 5 lb 10 oz

As an ex-midwife who has borne a son—my first, though I am twenty-nine—I have had experience of two different methods during labour. I can be objective in judging the value of the training for childbirth without pain and the necessity of taking an active part in the process of childbirth.

My labour started with the rupture of the membranes, followed an hour later by the appearance of contractions every twenty minutes. Three hours after the first contraction, I was at the nursing home, easily bearing the contractions which came now every ten minutes. I was already doing the quick breathing, which seemed to me to answer a need and which I did more easily than during my training. I was not prepared for the strong contractions which came every five minutes from 4 a.m. onwards, and the pains that I had to bear made me realize the necessity of not remaining passive.

From 4 till 8 a.m. I was alone in the labour ward. The midwife came from time to time, but I preferred solitude. I even sent my husband away, for he thought he could help by talking to me. I had not asked him to take part in the training. Alone and entirely absorbed in my confinement for four hours, I was amazed that I could control myself so well.

I felt relaxed, without a shadow of anxiety. I seemed to have a faint smile like that of a mezzo-soprano singer; at least this is what I felt. One is very proud to be in charge of the situation. Then my uterine contractions came more often and strongly. Mme D. found me in this condition, and I explained that I could not do without the quick breathing which seemed to put out the fire of the contractions.

At 4 a.m. I was given an injection of spasmalgine. It did not work until 8 a.m., but then I reacted too much. Between the pains I fell into a sort of comatose sleep, which I could not fight against, even though I wanted to control my contractions and get ready for them. At 8.30 the doctor examined me and said that the head was high and dilatation would not be easy; and this increased my inhibition. There was nothing alarming in what he said, but it proves how vulnerable we are. I felt prostrated. I begged them to wake me up because I was conscious of my state only when the contraction was at its height, and psychologically it was terribly tiring. What absolute reflex I had left enabled me, however, to do the quick breathing before the pain woke me up completely. Thanks to that, this last phase of my childbirth was very quick, to the surprise of the doctor, the midwife and my husband. It was the delivery which surprised me most, too. Being an ex-midwife, I remembered the average time this takes, and when, after three good efforts and two pushes that I did badly, the doctor said that the head, then the face, had appeared, I could not believe my ears.

The pleasant shock of my son's birth removed at least half of my uncontrollable desire to sleep. The unexpected effects of the spasmalgine were attributed to the fact that, before, I had only been treated by homoeopathy.

I am grateful for this method which makes childbirth without pain possible, and the doctors who make the extra effort of using it. I was in a position to judge the help it brought me by comparing the moments when I could use what I had learnt and the moments when I could not.

6

The Failures

THE argument that there should be no failures with a scientific method might be valid in mathematical matters. But the human being is essentially changeable, and is constantly influenced by external environment. This is why there are failures in C.W.P. Far from detracting from the method, they strengthen its principles. Those who do not understand this do not understand what C.W.P. is.

A distinction must be made between the various causes of failure. We will omit the medical and obstetrical causes. Each doctor can explain them to his patient before confinement, so that she knows what improvement she may expect from the method. But there are other important influences which may lead to failure.

The conditions themselves may be faulty. The training may be bad or incomplete. The maternity home may not be equipped for C.W.P., or the unit may not be sufficiently separated from the ordinary midwifery service. Several women may go through their confinement together in one ward. This will create an unpleasant atmosphere, reminiscent of hospital or nursing home—which implies illness. The place of childbirth must be called a 'maternity home', and must not seem like a hospital.

Uneducated or hostile staff may cause difficulties. When we started we saw this happening. Many times our trained women told us of adverse comment from hospital or nursing-home staff. 'You believe in C.W.P.? You'll soon see when the pains get bad.' Or, 'Don't bother about those stupid ideas. I know what I'm saying.' Or, 'It's only suggestion, and you know that's dangerous.'

And we hear of still greater stupidity. 'You must have a political slant for it to work. It operates best with the Slavs, badly for Westerners and not at all for the Latin races.'

The public has also been told that 'the method is dangerous to the child'. But according to statistics no method produces better results. Critics have even declared that psychoprophylaxis may have serious effects on women's psychology. Reports in this book refute such an idea. A section—fortunately very small—of the medical profession has had an adverse influence in a way quite out of keeping with medical ethics. Some doctors have outright denied the value of the method—for which they bear a heavy responsibility. The opposition has meant delay in its use and has been an important cause of some failures.

Sometimes inexperienced people use the method. C.W.P. cannot be improvised; it must be thoroughly studied and understood. It is a completely new form of education, and those who want to use it properly must enter into it with appropriate humility. Every experimenter who varies it according to his own personal ideas will cause distress. Women will suffer; failures will increase, and there will be doubt instead of confidence. If the method is applied strictly by trained, convinced people, failures should not exceed 10 per cent. This percentage should decrease as our knowledge grows.

FAILURE DUE TO THE WOMAN HERSELF

We may blame the woman, but possibly the teacher is responsible in that he has not early enough detected the factor which has a bad effect at childbirth. The few examples that we give indicate the instability of the cortical equilibrium that we try to achieve. The event which causes failure may be far past or recent, or may occur during confinement itself. Systematic studies of the failures, and comparison of our conclusion with that of the woman, will help us to learn more every day, and, as a result, to cut down the failures.

Confidence is the main factor making for success.

Mme C. Age: 26. Para. 2. 21 April, 1955. Girl 8 lb 14 oz
I wanted to give birth to my baby without pain. 'Wanted' is not perhaps the word I should use. Let us say, 'hoped'. At times I believed I could do this, but at others the fear of failure paralysed me. At the last minute I gave way, even though everything seemed with me—in particular, the exceptionally easy conditions of my confinement. Labour began at 3.30 a.m., and the baby was born at 6.32 a.m.

The end of my pregnancy was happy; I felt gay, much more active than usual, waking up with the spring. Above all there was the joy of waiting for a baby.

Eight days before the birth things started to go less well. I was nervous, a bit tired, discontented, although I continued to lead an active life as before. Perhaps it would have been better if I had not been warned that the confinement might take place before the expected date. I was impatient, and the last days of waiting seemed long.

When labour began early in the morning I was very surprised, I did not believe it at first. I was afraid of being wrong, and in any case I was very anxious, and—I do not know why—in a bad mood. My husband tried to cheer me up, and partially succeeded. But each time I had the chance of recovering my spirits, of pulling myself together during the confinement, I refused to do so.

I got ready to leave very carefully, without forgetting anything, and this helped me to calm down and to forget myself a bit. When I felt some contractions, I did the quick respiration, but managed only once to do it perfectly. But during the weaker contractions I did realize how effective the relaxation was.

I found out at the clinic that I was between three fingers and half dilated. I should have regained confidence as labour was already so far on—and I felt that I could manage it. It was during the contractions when I was between half and three-quarters dilated that I completely lost my grip. A wave of the same sensations as in my first confinement came over me, especially the terror of the delivery. I realized that it was time to pull myself together if I wanted to succeed at the most interesting and moving phase of the confinement. I was surprised to find how easy it was. And yet, because I was angry and disgusted with myself on account of my behaviour, I took shelter in failure.

I asked you, doctor, to anaesthetize me, remembering your remark that women who ask for this disappoint you. I wanted to spoil everything rather than half succeed. I was unhappy when I thought that you had really put me to sleep, but I still heard people's voices and gradually I recovered consciousness. I was still very afraid in spite of the urgent need that I felt to push. Your insistence and encouragement made me try timidly, and I was astonished that, in spite of my very small effort, something came of it. I started pushing again with a little more enthusiasm, although without conviction, and I felt that the second push was almost right. I did not want to see my baby born because I was sulking.

But I am no longer afraid of delivery. I feel ready to start again.

There is no need for fear. It is not painful. It is only a question of will-power, of effort, and it is so surprising and amazing to feel the progress of the baby that, once you have begun to make the effort, you cannot stop.

To conclude—I believe that I was very confused by the irregularity of the contractions from the start. The movements of the baby mingled with them or came in between them, and I had difficulty in distinguishing the real from the false contractions. I really did not take advantage of the moments of rest.

Anne was born yesterday. The day was unpleasant, but today I am happy. I feel well and, although I did not give birth quite 'without pain', I suffered very little and I could have avoided it. I was conscious when my baby was born, and that could not have happened without your help. This is very important to me. When I was anaesthetized for my first baby I did not mind very much. I indulged in the excuse of having too narrow a pelvis—as I had been told. Now that I have been trained I should have suffered morally if I had been anaesthetized again. I understand why you told me that I did not fail completely.

Mme M. Age: 33. Para. 2. 22 October, 1955. Boy 7 lb 5 oz

I have the reputation of being well belanced. Living among psychologists, I have often tried personality tests, and I have always been above normal. It is true that most of these tests are designed for the investigation of the grossest abnormalities. In addition, fourteen years of life in England taught me self-control in moderation. It did not create inhibitions in me as it does in the English, who practise self-control in large quantities from the first feeding bottle.

In spite of all this, it ended in a complete fiasco.

I had no anxiety before the confinement. Neither did I have any for my first labour, thirteen years ago, which I do not remember very well. I attended the lectures with interest, and I conscientiously did the exercises that the assistant taught me. I was happy at the thought of having the assistant beside me. I waited confidently, without doubting that everything would happen as predicted. I was alone at home, my husband being at the hospital, but I had the telephone number of the ambulance and I was very busy. I continued to work to the end, and I drove my car till two days before childbirth.

The pains started in the middle of the afternoon, very slight and irregular. I was afraid to go to the clinic too early, because I remembered waiting twenty-four hours in a clinic for the first childbirth. However, on the doctor's advice I went at about nine o'clock. At 9.30 p.m. I was one finger dilated. At about ten o'clock the pains were still irregular but increasing, and I started the quick breathing. They suddenly became very strong when the assistant arrived about 11.30 p.m. I realized I was not quite relaxed. Mme — reassured me, 'It will come.' The contractions were very frequent, but I relaxed gradually, and dealt with them in good time, warned by the assistant well before I felt them myself. Everything came on very quickly. I think I began to have pain when I was between half and three-quarters dilated, but the contractions were never completely painless.

I reasoned with myself continuously. I tried to relax, and when, at the end of a contraction, I looked for the arm of the assistant who held the oxygen mask it was for moral support. I never clutched her arm.

At 12.30 a.m., when the doctor arrived, I tried to joke, but another contraction and an intolerable pain quickly stopped my attempts at humour. I was very angry with myself. I was fighting against something I could not understand, which should not have happened.

I partly spoilt the delivery, but I was aware it was my fault, although I felt I was not consciously responsible for what happened during the first part of labour. I had great difficulty in resuming the deep breathing for the second push during a contraction, probably because of the half-sitting position which is, however, so comfortable for pushing.

I also had intense pins and needles in my legs, because of bad circulation, which troubled me a lot.

I greatly appreciated the remarks of the doctor during delivery. He was like Georges Briquet[1] at his best. I found this sports commentary very encouraging.

This is only a preliminary report. I really want to understand why I failed. I am sure that it was due to psychological causes, and that the only way to improve the techniques of childbirth without pain is to work out the psychological symptoms of pregnant women and their behaviour during childbirth.

Mme G. Age: 26. Para. 2. 17 April, 1954. Boy 6 lb 8 oz

I cannot say that I shall be brief. Words seem to me very important, making discussion, contact, persuasion—or exorcism—possible.

A confinement takes a woman, almost without an intermediate stage, to a quite different state. This causes shock, and she later tries to free herself in various ways—by confidences to her friends, thoughts

[1] A well-known radio sports commentator in France.

pondered in silence, and so on. You have asked me for a report. I will tell you what I have thought out in the nights when I could not sleep.

I cannot talk of my second confinement without mentioning the first. They were quite different, but they form a unit for me. I have compared them so much.

It was not really the fear of suffering which led me to try this experiment. It was for more positive reasons, which make my conclusions more complicated. Of course I faced my first childbirth apprehensively, but I realized that I was neither the first nor the last to go through it, and I wanted to get it over. At first I was more optimistic about the second one. It seemed natural that the 'running in' of the organs should make things easier.

I did not want to go through the hospital experience again—the screams of my neighbours, the light dazzling my eyes, the bed-pan under me much too soon, making the lumbar pains worse, because 'the more tired the woman, the better the labour', the scolding of the midwives, 'stimulants' which depressed me, etc. . . . Yet all this was not as bad as the ten following days stewing in bed, forbidden to get up and open the window even a little, and the feeling of being reduced to absolute silence, caught in pitiless machinery.

In the autumn I came across a series of articles in newspapers and various magazines. They were of different lengths, and used different arguments, but they were all more or less convinced. They seemed confirmation of my own conclusions: childbirth should be otherwise conducted. But words are, I thought, not enough. If I wanted to fight prejudice I must do more. I made up my mind to attempt this experiment myself.

My first childbirth was very baffling and began three weeks before term. I had a few sudden pains at long intervals in the pubic symphysis; then one evening at dinner violent pains, like colic, began and came oftener and oftener but stopped at about 3 a.m. There was nothing more until the next evening, when the same thing started again. As a precaution, I took some Epanal to calm me down. Indeed I do not really know what I took. But it was in vain. The next morning the doctor diagnozed two fingers dilatation. I arrived at the hospital at noon, though I was not to be delivered before 1 a.m. I heard absolutely inhuman screams. It was very upsetting but I promised myself I would not scream whatever happened—out of pride, and not to lose strength that was already impaired by lack of sleep. Of course, at the crucial moment, I was exhausted. I had no strength to breathe in the trilene mask. I was told to breathe deeply when my pain was bad, but each time it was too late, and it did not help.

I had no more strength to push either. I had promised myself I would see my baby appear, but I even forgot that he was going to be born. I was confused by the one wish not to scream. So I had a bitter feeling of frustration, which was only lessened by avidly reading my husband's books on obstetrics.

With the second pregnancy, the expected 'running in' was apparent. I had less nausea and little backache.

I was very interested in the training. My friends, who were doubtful at first, were gradually impressed by my confident attitude. I avoided talking about it to my doctor—a family friend who had categorically advised me to go to hospital for my first 'because one never knows', advice against which I violently revolted at the time.

Fifteen days and then eight days before my second confinement I had heavy falls in the garden. On Good Friday I felt a few contractions. At eleven o'clock I went to bed, and suddenly realized that they were close together—every seven minutes exactly. I was sleepy and too lazy to get up. I thought that it would be like the first time. My husband was worried, and consulted his encyclopaedia, looking for a symptom to convince me that I was wrong. He found one—the presence of 'blood-stained mucus'. Then I began to lose the waters and I got up quickly because nothing was ready. Labour had once more arrived three weeks before term.

We called the ambulance. After an hour it still had not come. We telephoned to the clinic, to you, doctor, to neighbours, but did not get a sound. There were no more trains, and we had no car.

I did not dare to count the minutes between contractions, I was so afraid of being delivered without a doctor and being torn—as I had heard my mother describe so often. I did not remember that the installation of an important telephone exchange, a mile away, might have upset our line. I let myself be overcome by an intolerable feeling of impotence. I tried hard to practise the quick breathing and relaxation, but did not succeed.

At about 2 a.m. the police ambulance came. At the clinic I found that I was only two fingers dilated. Of course, I had pain. I expected this to be like the first time, with fifteen hours, just as bad, in front of me. This made me more nervous. My worry only stopped an hour later when the doctor came, five minutes or so before delivery.

Perhaps my report should have been kept to these few lines. . . .

It is certain that rapid breathing is a help—perhaps I did not do it well enough to say to what extent—even if it is only as a diversion. And this time I had the joy of seeing my baby born. Also the clinic has an atmosphere of understanding and kindness down to the smallest detail, which made an enormous difference to me. At the hospital I counted the hours; here I do not even count the days.

But what is my conclusion about the method itself? The soil may be excellent and well sown, but the harvest can be completely spoiled by unexpected storms. It is necessary to wait and sow again.

This is my honest and grateful testimony to your method. For my third baby I shall follow it again, without hesitation or reservations, and I hope then not to remain dissatisfied.

Meanwhile, does it seem stupid to you that I want to finish the training by attending your last lecture and film?

Mme de M. Age: 32. Para. 4. 12 February, 1955. Boy

Here at last is the report that you asked me for—but first I want to express my gratitude, and tell you how much I hope that your wonderful undertaking will go on well.

You will find many of the impressions that I have already mentioned in our conversation. I apologize for the repetition. I did not send it to you before, because I thought that you might not want to bother with my experiences. I realized, the day before yesterday, that was not so, and that all the details that you are given help to build up knowledge. I hope that you will find some little thing which may help in these few lines. Here then are my main impressions—impressions confirmed by time. Already more than a month has passed.

My confinement, although very easy, was not perfect. It was a bit my fault, but much more the fault of circumstances. This baby was my fourth, and I did not want it very much. The memory of my previous confinements was much too clear. I felt, too, that I might be trying the new method like a game, for its novelty. I lacked faith and enthusiasm, though I did feel confidence in those who looked after me, and also some pride—not to appear too hopeless to them. In these conditions my training was very bad—even worthless. I remembered what was explained to me but never trained myself. This was a mistake. Practice was the thing I missed most during dilatation, and this was the least brilliant part of my labour. The rest with you, doctor, went fairly well. Delivery is an act, something which fills your mind and body. This part of childbirth seems to me easier than dilatation, which becomes active only through will-power. Delivery demands an effort, a very great physical effort, but if it is well done it is completely painless. After it one has a feeling of completeness and well-being. It is an infinitely pleasant state of healthy tiredness—rather what one feels at the end of a climb when the peak is reached. I was satisfied with my effort, and this feeling prevailed over all the others—even the joy of having a son.

I have only one regret. I already have four children, and shall not be able to examine properly the beautiful prospect that I have glimpsed.

The effect of childbirth without pain continues well after the confinement itself. I never felt so calm and relaxed as after this fourth birth. One feels fully alive—and for that, too, I can never thank you enough.

7

Foreign Women Giving Birth in France

THIS chapter answers two frequently raised questions: is child-birth without pain applicable to any type of woman, or to any temperament?

Like all scientific methods, it cannot and should not discriminate. Latin races can benefit from it as well as Nordic, Asiatic or European; the white woman as well as the coloured.

The physiology of the uterine muscle is the same in all climates. The differences are caused by the conditions in which women live, their upbringing and the atmosphere at their confinement. Though the basic rules of the method must be strictly observed everywhere, the method of application may vary. The doctor in Peking works differently from a Portuguese doctor in Lisbon; an American doctor in New York differently from a Swiss doctor in Geneva. In every country, different conditions influence the woman's behaviour in relation to confinement.

This chapter contains reports from women in other countries. Others who have had babies according to the method of childbirth without fear evolved by the English doctor, G. Dick Read, comment on the difference. They prefer childbirth without pain, which remains a wonderful experience of activity.

Childbirth without pain crowned their efforts and made them realize their own personalities. 'I am proud of myself. I have fully succeeded in my childbirth' is a perfectly justified boast, since child-birth has become their task.

Mrs. Stanley Geist, American. Age: 30. Para. 2. 28 November, 1952.
   Boy
My confidence in the method of childbirth without pain was mixed with some doubt. I had read that such a confinement should be in some way a mystical phenomenon, or related to auto-suggestion.

Being too rational (if not reasonable) to take up this sort of spiritual exercise, I thought that in applying myself to a physical and mental régime of training I could expect at best a lessening of the pains. Now, after my second confinement (the first to use this method), I know that it is not a matter of mysticism but quite simply of physiology and of a mind cleared, by detailed training, of ignorance and doubt, and the fears which they produce. I could never have believed that childbirth could be so easy. My amazement is shared by my husband who, having been at the birth of my two children is grateful to Dr. — for having saved him this second time from the panic, the screams, the miseries, which characterized the first labour.

Several days before the expected date I was warned one afternoon by a slight discharge that the moment was nearer than I thought. The doctor advised me on the telephone to go to the clinic that evening.

My mind and body were in good form (although I was a bit tired by going out too much). I had attended two lectures given by the doctor and some training classes at the assistant's. Even with this small training I should probably not have been afraid of labour; but I might have kept some disturbing doubts mainly about the physiology. And in spite of what I had learned, I did not believe that I should have only a few unpleasant hours. I was resigned to worse. I waited impatiently for the birth of my baby. The price to pay in physical suffering (which I do not stand well) did not seem to me too much.

My case was ready and I went to the hairdresser. I had dinner quietly at home, and then left for the clinic with my husband. The midwife's examination showed that I was only two fingers dilated and that I should probably not be delivered before the morning. Rather than be bored all night in the labour ward waiting for the contractions, I left, after having arranged my things, to spend the evening at the cinema. At midnight—nothing; at one o'clock still nothing. But I went back to the clinic to sleep.

About 3 a.m., I felt the first contractions. They were slight, like menstrual pains. They stopped about 5 a.m. and did not start again until 10.30 a.m.—a little stronger. At three o'clock I tried the method of relaxation and breathing learnt at the assistant's for the first time. They were perfectly successful, but this was not very convincing since the contractions were not really very strong. A second try at 10.30 a.m., with complete suppression of the pain, gave me a great surprise.

I thought: 'It's all right for the present. Later we shall see. It can't be so easy.'

The doctor arrived, ruptured the membranes and gave me an injection to speed up the rhythm of the contractions. During the next three hours they became quicker and much stronger. At the beginning of each I started to breathe and to relax properly, always with the expected result: immediate and complete relief of pain. 'Almost always' would be more exact. Several times I missed the beginning (often hardly perceptible) of a contraction, not knowing how to recognize it, and, during the few moments which passed before I caught up and synchronized the rhythm of my quick breathing, I realized what in other conditions the pain could have been like. The doctor helped me to synchronize the breathing with the contractions until I knew how to do it perfectly myself. Once, when the doctor was not there for a short time, I was surprised by a particularly strong contraction and I suddenly tensed myself instead of relaxing. An intense pain took my breath away. I panicked, lost control of my breathing and let out one of those cries like a suffering animal which punctuate a traditional labour. The doctor came back, and again controlled my timing, so that the following contractions, which were stronger and stronger, caused me no pain at all.

At a certain moment the rhythm of the contractions changes from

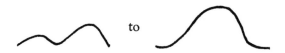

When the change occurred, I had some difficulty in resynchronizing my breathing rhythm. I think it would be advisable, during the training, to dwell as much on this change as on the one which precedes delivery.

The doctor, my husband and I spent most of these three hours talking quietly as if we had been at home. The conversation was periodically interrupted: not by pains and screams but by the breathing and relaxation exercises which took their place. My breathing had dried my lips, and they brought me some water. It would seem a small detail, but it was very important, because such details made up a general (and essential) atmosphere of relaxation, and the feeling that I was not there to undergo a test but to bring a child into the world as naturally as possible. What worried me most of all was that I was hungry.

Towards the end of this period, the contractions had become very strong. I thought: 'Here we are at last. Until now it has been a game. Now we begin work seriously—that is painfully. In a few hours everything will be over.' But no, it was already the end. Between two contractions, the doctor explained to me how I must now push and breathe deeply instead of quickly. I had another difficult moment especially from the relaxation point of view, in changing over from the last contraction to the first push of the baby downwards. I felt a sudden prolonged pressure in the region of the anus, with a momentary sensation of confusion, doubt and fright. But it was quickly dispelled by the doctor, who insisted that I should relax and showed me a new respiratory rhythm. I pushed, breathing deeply. All went well. The pressure continued, but without being painful.

They brought me oxygen to strengthen the last movements of delivery. I knew, thanks to the doctor's lectures, what was happening. The oxygen mask did not frighten me at all, and the fact that the mask is made of transparent material greatly lessened the instinctive repulsion at the idea of something on my face. But the unusual feeling of the mask covering my mouth and nose gave me the idea that I did not know how to breathe properly—or could not. I was confused by this idea, and no longer clearly understood the doctor's instructions, or clearly remembered the lessons learnt. I began to counteract the efforts of my own body. Once more I lost control of my breathing. My muscles contracted; I moved my head and arms about; I felt acute pain. And once again it was the insistent voice of the doctor that indicated the breathing rhythm which I must keep up and reminded me of the muscular relaxation, and so cut short the pain, as well as this futile performance.

I kept on pushing. The doctor announced, while controlling the rhythm of my pushing and encouraging me: 'Here is the head . . . the forehead . . . the eyes . . . the nose . . . the chin . . . the shoulders. . . . .' I looked on, amazed. Here, in fact, was my baby who—strange and unbelievable fact—came out of me. And here, as he came out, were inexpressible feelings of physical pleasure, of well-being, of liberation, of deliverance, of euphoria. He was hardly delivered when I heard him cry. The doctor held him up for me to see. It was a boy. Perfectly clear-minded and awake, I expressed my happiness in almost correct French. To my husband who came to congratulate me, I whispered (not wishing to offend the doctor): 'It is not true that one feels *no* pain. I felt something once—when they gave me the oxygen mask.' I realized afterwards the implication of such a remark.

While they cut the cord and put the baby's binder on, I made myself comfortable and talked to my husband and the doctor.

I was a bit afraid of the contractions which precede and accompany the delivery of the placenta, but everything went easily and without difficulty. I waited for the 'inevitable' post-natal troubles after a second confinement. Should I suffer from depression, or physical and moral exhaustion? Nothing of the kind. Meanwhile, I was happy, though a little stupefied. I felt well. I was hungry. I asked immediately for something to eat, but without much hope of getting anything. After all, it was a sort of operation that I had just gone through. The reply was unexpected! 'Why not? You have not had an anaesthetic.' They brought me a good lunch. I ate well and I slept until the evening.

I waited during the hours and days following for the post-natal euphoria to give way to an 'inevitable' state of nervous depression. Nothing. It was almost exasperating. I felt so flourishing that I was weary of days with nothing to do. I got impatient. I wanted to go home. I consoled myself with my baby, who was beside me. I had been deprived of that pleasure after my first confinement, but now I recognize that it is of immense value.

Mme Arensburg, Argentinian. Age: 22. Para. 2. 4 July, 1955. Girl 6 lb 3 oz

For myself and my husband my second childbirth without pain was a wonderful proof of conditioning, especially as I saw Mme C. only four days before childbirth and I was not trained at all. Mme C. was in charge of training for my first confinement and of the classes which I attended at the P. Rouquès clinic.

I had a bad conscience up to the last minute because of my negligence. I also thought that the physical factors which handicapped me for my first childbirth would handicap me again. (I had the scar of an extra-uterine pregnancy and a very sensitive lumbo-sacral area.) But the facts turned out quite differently.

On Sunday night, when I was with friends, I felt three contractions, a quarter of an hour apart; but, as they did not continue, I put them down to tiredness. Afterwards I spent a peaceful night and day. At 4.55 p.m. on the Monday afternoon, I had another contraction, which I still attributed to fatigue, since my term was between 10 and 15 July.

But I noticed at 5.15 p.m. that I had contractions too often for the beginning of labour (every three minutes), so I telephoned the doctor, who advised me to come to the clinic for observation.

I got ready to go quite quietly, left my eleven-months-old baby in the hands of a responsible person, and departed with my husband. During the journey by taxi I was very relaxed and happy, and I quietly did the slow deep breathing, which was sufficient. I thought I was at the beginning of labour and that on arrival I should have an injection to lessen the frequency of contractions.

How surprised and glad we were when the midwife after examining me said I was fully dilated! It was seven o'clock. We laughed with my husband and wondered how and when I had got through the whole first part of labour. Logically, as soon as I knew I was fully dilated, my respiratory needs changed, and I adopted the quick respiration without realizing it. This too made us laugh.

I was taken into the labour ward at 7.20 p.m. The doctor and Mme C. came at 7.30 p.m.; and at 7.40 p.m. after two pushes, my little girl was born. Something upset me at the end of the first push and I lost control for a few seconds. I felt that I could not push, that my will did not respond. But when the doctor and my husband said, 'But the head is here. Look' and I bent forward and saw it, all my inhibition disappeared. I pushed once more, and it was all over. My baby was almost out, and the doctor gave her to me to hold.

In the happiness and excitement, I had completely forgotten that we wanted a girl. Only when I heard my husband exclaim happily, 'It's a girl!' did I react and looked quickly to be sure of our luck.

We were really impressed by the method of childbirth without pain. If any doubts remained after my first confinement—doubts which were, even so, personal ones—now I could say that, with this method, one could have a baby every day.

Mme Nelson, Italian. Age: 23. Primip. 6 February, 1954. Boy

I write my impressions of childbirth without pain, in the hope that they will bring confidence and optimism to future mothers—especially in Italy where I do not know if this method has ever been used.

It is a wonderful and uplifting experience. I hope that in my country the new method will gain the popularity it is getting here, where interest and enthusiasm increase every day.

The first time that I saw my doctor, I was greatly impressed. His explanations introduced me to a world of knowledge and opportunities which had been unknown to me until then. First of all, there was a new training for the mind, which in childbirth without pain becomes the most important factor. The woman's brain must be cleared of a past of prejudices, fear and obscurantism. A whole programme of physical training had to be followed with discipline and goodwill. 'Like a real athlete who trains himself for a race,' said the doctor. And in fact, the two essentials in childbirth without pain are to learn how to breathe and to control each muscle in the body by controlling the reflexes.

I started training at the beginning of the eighth month. Mme C., a physiotherapist, took the practical classes fortnightly and the doctor gave the theoretical lectures. I trained myself every night as hard as I could.

It is really extraordinary to see how from theory one passes to practice. Training enables such a high level of perception that one is able to do the exercises with the greatest precision even before the beginning of contractions and to time the depth of the breathing with the strength of contractions.

My husband's help was useful during this phase of preparation. He gave practical and moral support which was very important—a bit like the crowd's excited encouragement for the athlete.

I felt this even more with Dr. V. during the delivery, the most tiring and difficult part of labour, but in childbirth without pain also the most exciting. Here really is a triumph for the woman. She is conscious all the time, and absolute arbiter of her labour. In the culminating moments mother and baby are united in a unique and final effort to open the last passage into life. It is in these last moments that the voice and words of the doctor raise the already wonderful experience to an exciting pitch.

I shall never forget the last hours spent in waiting for our baby. The first real contractions began unexpectedly at seven o'clock in the evening, and, as the doctor had warned me, with an interval of twenty minutes between each. I lay on the bed, gently massaging my stomach to relieve the pain, and began slow deep breathing each time. This always had the expected effect. Little by little I learnt to anticipate the contractions which were becoming more frequent all the time. I did not want to begin quick respiration yet, so as not to tire myself. As I had been advised, I kept it for the proper time. This time was not slow in coming.

About ten o'clock, on the advice of the doctor whom my husband had telephoned, I went to the clinic. I was nervous, anxious and happy at the great event that I was going to experience and also keyed up by a sort of strong curiosity. I was taken to the labour ward, and there the impressive wait started and the moments ticked by. I was determined not to let myself miss the least thing. While I was talking quietly to Mme C. and my husband, who were helping me, all the nerves and muscles of my body and my brain were tense, ready for action.

When, after the first examination, the midwife had said that I should probably have to wait the whole night, I felt disappointed. But membranes broke a little later and immediately everything speeded up. The contractions followed at short intervals, one every two minutes and much stronger. The slow deep breathing was no longer enough, and I started the quick shallow breathing—at the end of each contraction a long breath in.

From one special small aid I derived great benefit. At a given moment Mme C. lightly massaged my stomach round and round, and from this I felt greater relief than when I did it myself. In this way I could relax more completely during the contractions. This fact may seem insignificant, but a woman's smallest experience can perhaps improve this technique, which in France is only two years old.

Time passed quickly. Every now and then I looked at my wrist watch. Then suddenly I saw the doctor beside me. It was the decisive moment, that of full dilatation and the beginning of delivery. The full team was there—Mme C., the doctor, my husband. At a new contraction I raised myself, stopped breathing and took a good hold of the stirrup bars. The doctor's voice ordered: 'There now! Push, push. Stronger, again, again, again. That's fine! Relax!'

I let myself fall back, breathing quickly, making myself relax completely. But my brain kept on working strongly so as to maintain a high level of perception and not to lose precious control. This is the time when you recover, after immense effort, between two contractions. To my confidence there was now added a great feeling of triumph. The two months' training were producing expected results. Although, sometimes, in the period of training, I had had momentary doubts, I felt now, with a wonderful certainty, that I had learned the power of serene control of the birth of our baby minute by minute and without pain.

Three, four, five times the contractions started again, and I raised myself, gripped the bars, stopped breathing and concentrated all my physical strength in a single effort. And suddenly, during my effort,

I heard the voice of the doctor, giving me instructions, encouraging me and telling me step by step how labour was progressing.

The baby's head pressed on the perineum. The order was to stop pushing, to relax completely, just to breathe strongly to avoid any tear. And here was the head . . . the eyes . . . the nose . . . a shoulder . . . the other shoulder. Bach's second Brandenburg concerto greeted our son's entry into the world. Our son!

Accompanied by this sublime, triumphant music came the first cry, the first unconscious salute to the life that I had given. It may be surprising that music was played in the labour ward at such a time. It was perhaps the first occasion that such a thing had happened, but one day I had told the doctor I wanted this and he said, 'Why not?' Anything which might help or encourage the woman is welcomed for the development of the technique.

I should finally like to pay homage to the great scientist, Pavlov. His experiments on conditioned reflexes have made the scientific development of childbirth without pain possible.

Effects of C.W.P. on the Parents, the Child and their Activities

TRADITIONALLY the husband's behaviour changes during his wife's pregnancies and confinements. During the first pregnancy he is attentive and thoughtful, though he does not know what to do to help. He is moved and proud, and shows his superiority; and he takes part in the creation of a passive attitude in his wife, who feels like a little girl protected by her mother and husband.

Sometimes, towards the end of pregnancy, the wife appears deformed, almost ugly, to her husband. He may make any excuse for leaving her alone. She is tired he says, or she might be if she goes out, and he thinks of her almost as if she were ill or an invalid.

When labour begins, the husband usually keeps out of the way. He is worried as soon as it starts, and he has only one aim—to get his wife to the clinic. He takes part in the general upset, the last feverish moments, but he is very glad when the doctor tells him to go and smoke a few cigarettes in the waiting-room or garden. Some husbands, wanting to relieve their wives' tortures, are present at the labour, but with tense faces, horrified by the women's screams.

Childbirth itself is rarely endured by the husband, who turns pale and has to be sent out of the room quickly. In fact, the woman, feeling lowered, humiliated and ugly, prefers her mother to her husband. He is frightened and shocked, and is thankful to run away. He waits for his wife's delivery—which is as much his own. He feels guilty, and plays a useless and completely passive rôle. As soon as childbirth ends, the unrelieved tension under which he has lived for several hours is suddenly released.

In the next pregnancies the picture changes, and this the more so the more there are. The husband is much less attentive; he no longer fusses. He leaves his wife more easily, and she finds herself alone, cut adrift or in unkind hands. Judged by the husband's behaviour, his sense of guilt and responsibility decreases with the number of pregnancies. Indifferent, he comes to regard pregnancy and childbirth as a habit.

This depressing, almost degrading situation for the husband tends to disappear completely with C.W.P. It seems that the husbands themselves have quickly realized this. Women often say at their first visit, 'I have come to see you because my husband wants me to try this experiment.' We soon came to realize that husbands should play an important part in the training and confinement. This is a matter of observation and simple logic.

The behaviour of the pregnant woman is primarily influenced by the people she lives with. Their unsympathetic attitude is caused by general ignorance. The best solution would be to educate everybody, but, as this is not at present possible, we have limited our efforts to the family, which is the smallest unit of society.

We begin with the husband. If he cannot attend the lectures, the wife will tell him what she learns, so as to revise her own knowledge and to discover the gaps in it. More and more, interested husbands are coming with their wives to the lectures, which are developing into exciting subjects of friendly conversation. Interest increases all the time. The husband stimulates his wife, encourages her, comforts her, foresees her difficulties and urges her to discuss them with the doctor. He helps every day by avoiding all incidents which might harm her—unpleasant conversation, argument, unwise books, etc. He becomes the doctor's active collaborator, makes his wife practise her exercises and controls her breathing or neuromuscular relaxation. He has a part to play, and is fully conscious of it, carrying it out with enthusiasm and intelligence.

The passive gives way to the active. It is a victory, too, for the man who is freed from his feeling of guilt. He assesses his responsibilities, and rises to them. Stronger emotional bonds are created between the couple and are consecrated through childbirth. The husband is impressed by his wife's dignity. It is not necessary to drive him from the labour ward, because there, too, he plays his part and participates in the birth of his child. The act of birth takes on beauty in his eyes. A communion is established and strengthened by the first cry of the baby, who no longer seems to spring only from the hard painful work of the mother, but from the couple's united effort.

Even in cases of unwanted pregnancy, we have seen couples overflowing with happiness at the birth. Childbirth without pain was at first the woman's victory; it quickly became that of the couple.

There is another factor—inner peace. The calmness that the woman finds—thanks to the training during pregnancy—and the harmony with her husband affect the whole family and especially the other children. The parents understand them better, and the feeling of jealousy in any child at the birth of a brother or sister lessens and tends to disappear. The training of the parents has been successful, and the children themselves derive benefit from it. Many family quarrels and misunderstandings are avoided. Knowledge and its application result in joy and happiness. The man and woman become equal in the most important act—creating life.

There is one point to be stressed because of its social importance. We have seen women who, shortly after giving birth without pain, were pregnant again. All of them have said this: 'If I had not had childbirth without pain, I should not have wanted another pregnancy, nor would my husband.'

So we think that C.W.P., in changing the attitude of the couple, can create one means of dealing with the great problem of abortion—a means which the Government should not neglect. Childbirth without pain does not end with the birth. It extends into the most varied fields of activity of both parents. We leave the reader to discover other remote effects through the following passages from letters. They are the replies to our circular sent to each woman who has given birth without pain asking permission to publish her account.

Mme Fragnaud. Age: 29 Primip. 18 November, 1955. Boy 6lb 14 oz.
   Report written by the husband
   When we saw the doctor on the seventeenth at 3 o'clock, he led us to believe that things would happen quite quickly. My wife was one finger dilated. We left the doctor's and went shopping, and at 5.30 p.m. we went on to the cinema. My wife had only very weak contractions, and she did not need to control them.

We returned home at 7.30 p.m., and dined quietly at about 9 o'clock. While we were getting ready for bed, my wife had a fairly strong contraction. She did not have time to control it at the beginning with quick breathing, so she had some bad moments. Exactly ten minutes later, she had another contraction, which was very acute, but using the famous quick respiration, she stood it perfectly well. Until about 10 o'clock, the contractions came every five to six minutes. My wife controlled them very well every time because she did the breathing as soon as they began.

At 10 o'clock we left for the clinic. During the journey I had to stop four times to allow my wife to control her contractions. She was put straight away into the labour ward, and I helped her until the assistant arrived at about 11.30 p.m. Dilatation was then about two fingers, and the contractions were coming regularly every three or four minutes. They lasted about two minutes and were particularly strong. Their strength, according to the assistant and the midwife, was much greater than normal; but my wife was well in control of herself. She remained calm and relaxed and stood them well. She then wanted to start pushing; but about seven years ago she had an electro-coagulation, and her cervix was thick and dilated too slowly compared with the contractions. So the midwife gave her an injection of methionate of magnesium to soften the cervix.

At 1.45 a.m. she was three fingers dilated, and then, in half an hour, went from a half to three quarters-dilated. At 2.45 a.m., she was fully dilated, and delivery started. I was still with her, and was helping her when she pushed. The baby presented as a right posterior, the head badly flexed. After only four pushes he became free and crossed the bony pelvis. Labour then took longer. About ten pushes were needed to make him turn and extend his head. The passage through the perineum then went normally, and, when the baby's head appeared, three pushes were enough to deliver him completely. The delivery lasted altogether thirty-five minutes, and needed seventeen pushes.

During this time my wife kept complete control. Only two pushes were incomplete and one spoilt, because of bad breathing which made her short of breath. The same evening she sat on the end of her bed and moved her legs. The following morning she got up, walked round the room three times without any help and did not feel at all tired.

Throughout labour my wife did not cry or groan at all. Her face was never tense; it was relaxed, and many times her eyes met mine and she smiled. What unforgettable joy to see one's baby come into the world with his mother smiling. Did she not say to the doctor while her baby was coming out, 'Oh doctor, it's wonderful', and, a few minutes later, 'I should like to start again to do better still'? What convincing proof of the complete success of childbirth without pain!

This account would not be complete if it ended here. To make a success of childbirth without pain, the woman must, throughout pregnancy, live in a pleasant atmosphere and with people who believe in the method. Sceptics should be firmly kept out of the way because they create doubt and mistrust. The husband should see to this. His part is very important. He and his wife should be good friends between whom perfect understanding and unbreakable confidence exist. It is not enough just to attend the lectures, and to go four times to the assistant's. The husband must keep an eye on his wife, make her do her exercises regularly every day and keep up her morale.

Mme Fragnaud adds: I should like to add a footnote to my husband's report. If I made a success of childbirth, I owe it mostly to him— to his optimism and perseverence in making me work and giving me confidence in myself. The achievement was the result of the collaboration of the doctor, my husband and, of course, myself.

This child is the fruit of a wonderful experience. I hope that all couples will in future have similar joy.

Mme Juquin. Age: 24 Para. 2. 18 July, 1955. Girl 7 lb 5 oz

My first confinement was normal but painful. Dilatation took twenty hours; delivery, three-quarters of an hour. For our second baby we decided to use childbirth without pain. I was greatly relieved that I should not suffer. Although this second birth was coming much sooner after the first than we should have wished, the method opened a stimulating prospect. I was going to do something more than the first time to help my baby come into the world.

Throughout the pregnancy I was thinking of the birth with a new interest. My husband made a great effort to come with me to the lectures which were at a particularly difficult time for him.

I started the lectures very late, in the eighth month of my pregnancy, because I was taking exams, and I could attend the doctor's first and fourth lectures only. The assistant, Mme X., whom I saw four times, explained the rest to me.

I was convinced from the beginning of the value of the method. From my first confinement I had remembered that, during labour, my pains were prolonged and increased by impatience, tenseness and ignorance; that efforts in delivery suppressed the pain, but that this effort needed to be directed and regulated to avoid useless exhaustion. The special number of the *Revue de la Nouvelle Médecine* and Colette Jeanson's book gave me a good introduction to the method.

The training helped me a lot. I did and improved my exercises every day, so strengthening my confidence. I was happy to work with my husband. His presence and help were also very precious to me at my confinement.

On 18 July, at about 11 p.m., I felt a very slight colic which I put down to some iced drinks that I had had during the day. The heat had been overpowering. Soon others followed—more violent. I attached little importance to them for several reasons. I had found a plausible explanation for them; and I remembered from my first childbirth localized pain in the back and slow and very gradual dilatation. Pains as long and as close together could only mean the end of dilatation.

My husband insisted that I was beginning labour. But I obstinately refused to believe it. About midnight the pains became unbearable. I groaned and lost control of myself more and more. On my husband's advice, I at last forced myself to relax, to do the quick breathing and to find out the exact nature of the colic. I gained control again when I first felt the need to push—very weak. From that moment there was no more doubt. What I felt fell into place in the scheme which I had learned at the lectures. I became calm again, and felt the advance of labour without suffering.

The contractions came every two or three minutes. We got a taxi in a hurry. During the journey I did the quick respiration. At every contraction I felt a desire to push. As soon as we arrived at the clinic, I lost the waters. The midwife examined me, sent me to the labour ward and telephoned the doctor.

He arrived a quarter of an hour later. I had felt the desire to push more strongly and more often—two or three times during each contraction. The contractions had made me breathless, and I had some difficulty in maintaining the rhythm of respiration. But my husband had encouraged me continually, and, thanks to him, I had waited for the doctor calmly and without making a mistake.

When he came in, my first thought was: 'At last. I am going to be able to push!' Delivery was very quick. In one push, my baby came down on to the perineum. I had the joy of feeling him descend. It was a sensation of considerable pressure but no pain. 'Do not push any more. Relax.' This was the most difficult moment. I managed to relax only with an effort, because the joy of feeling my baby so near and the pressure he exerted on my muscles made me push. This time again it was my husband who helped me. 'Relax completely,' he said, and I obeyed him.

The doctor announced that he was delivering the baby's face. 'Here is the forehead, the eyes, the nose, the mouth.' I clearly felt the head free itself. 'Another little push for the shoulders. There. Relax.'

I felt the first shoulder come out; then the second and the arm touching my body. The chest came out slowly by itself, and I could see my baby even before knowing its sex. I saw it open its mouth, move and put out its arms.

When it was completely delivered and had cried, they gave it to me, and I had the great joy of feeling its warm, moist little body in my hands. It was a girl. She weighed 7 lb 5 oz.

All this happened in a very calm atmosphere. My husband and I were relaxed and happy, amazed that my delivery had been so easy. We talked about it for several hours before he went home. I was not tired because I had not suffered, and I had had such sweet and pleasant feelings. I slept well, and got up two days later.

From this experience which we went through together, we have drawn several conclusions:

1. The method proved itself once more in my case. From the moment that I realized what was happening in me and controlled myself, I did not suffer.

2. But it is important to realize exactly when one is at the beginning of labour. I am not proud of having spoilt that part. I was not aware of the first phases, since I had no painful sensations during most of the dilatation. I should have remembered that two confinements in the same woman can be completely different.

3. It is a great joy for husband and wife together to accomplish an act important for both of them. My husband gave me considerable help by his presence, energy and constant encouragement. This birth has united us more closely.

The husband's point of view:

At the time of my wife's first confinement, in June 1954, I was abroad. I came home as quickly as possible, but could only reach the clinic a few hours after our daughter's birth. I had a strange painful feeling which for several hours spoilt the joy of fatherhood. Since everything was already done when I arrived, and this event, although so much ours, happened without me, I felt as though there were a separation, a rift, between us. I did not feel that I had really contributed to the birth of our child. My wife had lived through the most important experience without me. My child seemed a stranger to me. Of course, this unpleasant feeling did not last long. But today I still feel I have missed something which could have, which should have, been valuable in our life together.

Our second child was born without pain in July 1955. I will describe the event under four headings.

The decision: We had been aware for a long time of the existence of childbirth without pain and its remarkable results in Russia, China and France. We would have adopted it for our first child, if we had not then lived in West Germany. Here a professor of obstetrics asserted that he had only heard childbirth without pain mentioned in a one-page article in a magazine like *Paris Match*.

A friend from Cologne wrote to me: 'When I explained it to him and told him how widely the method is used in France, he replied with a doubtful smile: "A Russian method! Besides," he said, "no one has ever studied it, even out of curiosity. We rely on the good old methods."'

A strange conception of science and of the medical profession.

When we learnt that my wife was pregnant for the second time, we were in Paris. We immediately decided to try childbirth without pain. We knew nothing about the principles of the method, and had only a few limited ideas from school on Pavlov. Nevertheless, neither my wife nor I had any doubts, and we knew several friends who had given birth without pain by using this method.

People's reactions were not favourable.

Our doctor: 'You can always try. I have not studied the method nor seen the film, but several of my patients have asked me for this sort of confinement.'

A neighbour (close friend of the doctor): 'Childbirth without pain? Bah! it is entirely psychological, the Coué method.'

My mother-in-law (letter to her daughter): 'What you tell me of childbirth without pain is very interesting. I suppose that it consists of natural childbirth, which I read an article about: gymnastics, relaxation. Unless it is childbirth with injections.'

My father: 'A lot of expense and time wasted. It is a bad moment to go through. Don't let us make a drama of it. It would be better for you to prepare for your exams than for childbirth without pain.'

The training: Before starting the training itself, my wife read during the winter:

The special number of the *Revue de la Nouvelle Médecine* (too technical to be understood by non-specialists, but very interesting because of the number of case histories).

The book by Colette Jeanson (easily understood, certainly very attractive for a woman; but the poetic enthusiasm and some passages with a philosophical tendency do not conceal the shortcomings in descriptions and explanations. Therefore it cannot replace the training).

My wife started training very late—in June—and in unfavourable conditions. She was just about to take two parts of her degree. I had just sat for the written part of my exam, and we went through weeks of insomnia and anxiety. I could attend only one of the doctor's lectures and two of the assistant's classes. But my wife kept me in touch, and I helped her to do the exercises three times a day.

This co-operative training for childbirth not only suppressed the unpleasant feeling of which I spoke earlier—that every man has felt in similar circumstances—but it created new bonds. At the moment when my worries tended to make me withdraw into myself, to isolate myself and work on my own, our daily exercise gave me the feeling of discovering more and more about my wife's body and mind; created a new intimacy. The training for childbirth without pain strengthens the affection and mutual understanding of the couple. Between two of my oral exams I even managed to go to the assistant's lecture.

I add: that this serious training is necessary even for a woman convinced from the beginning of the efficacy of the method; that the husband's participation in this training is necessary. The way that my wife's confinement proceeded shows this.

The surprise: On 18 July, we had dinner very late. As soon as we were in bed, my wife, as on every night, did her exercises. At about 11 o'clock she felt violent colic. I immediately thought, 'This is it. You are going into labour'. But my wife replied, 'Oh no, certainly not. They are not contractions at all,' and thought the pain was due to an iced drink, which, quite unusually for her, she had had with the meal. If my wife had been a primip. I should have told her to start the exercises for childbirth, but I trusted in her experience.

But this experience was deceptive. Two confinements do not necessarily resemble one another. The assistant had told my wife so, but I think it would be a good thing to insist very strongly on this point during training.

One can feel pains in the back for the first child, and colic in the stomach for the second. A multip. should not be conditioned according to the first confinement, and should be taught how to detect contractions.

My wife suffered for a time; and this pain, which was almost continual—because it was, in fact, the last phase of dilatation, the whole of the first part having given no pain—was becoming intolerable. For a few minutes I saw what a woman can be like when she bears a baby in pain. It is horrible. My wife twisted about, half-unconscious, and repeated, 'It hurts. It hurts.'

I had a lot of difficulty in calming her. I had to scold her severely to get her to listen to me. Then, making her do the exercises automatically, I helped her to gain command of herself. Watch in hand, we timed the duration and frequency of the contractions—one every three minutes. I regulated her breathing. Suddenly, she sat up. In spite of her drawn features and still-haggard eyes, her face shone: 'I felt something pushing,' she said. 'I am going to give birth immediately. Let's get ready quickly.' From the time when she pulled herself together, my wife suffered no more and clearly followed everything that took place.

The success: When we arrived at the clinic my wife was fully dilated. I helped her to regulate her breathing while waiting for the doctor. We felt amazingly calm and relaxed. Once my wife took hold of my hand and squeezed it very strongly, tensing herself. I said to her, 'That's just the opposite of what you must do.' Immediately she relaxed completely.

The doctor arrived quickly, and my wife could then push. There again the value of the exercises showed itself. In her haste, she pushed anyhow at first, without having thought about breathing. The doctor immediately said: 'No.' I intervened. 'You have forgotten to breathe and hold it.' 'Ah! Yes, that's true,' she said and again, with great concentration, she did the exercise she had spoilt. This was a good thing. The baby, a girl of 7 lb 5 oz, came out with one single push. The end of delivery was very easy. We did not hear a single scream. The doctor joked. The nurses had hardly woken up. Taking our baby, my wife said, 'My darling'; then, 'It's wonderful.' To appear unmoved, I said, 'How ugly it is.' But I was thinking the opposite, of course.

One more detail: my wife had difficulty in taking hold of the stirrup bars to push. I gave her my hand, and she delivered our baby clutching me with all her strength.

Conclusion: I hope that this brief account, added to my wife's report, speaks for itself. Is not the progress of this particular birth excellent justification for the method? It shows that the main thing is to be well prepared and to control oneself. And so ends the old curse. Woman now gives birth without pain.

I emphasize the husband's collaboration. I believe that this confinement shows how some of a married couple's problems may be solved. Our second child was not planned, but, throughout the training—with patience and hard work—we wanted it. Thanks to the method, procreation is not a brief and single act, but creation prolonged by mutual effort. Finally, this method of childbirth seems to me not only to liberate women—who are no more slaves of the so-called 'inevitable' pain—but also partly to resolve the problem of freedom and necessity in marriage. It emphasizes the conscious work, will-power and intelligence of both partners in procreation.

Mme Cohen. Para. 2. 31 October, 1954. Girl 7 lb 15 oz

There is an essential difference between my emotional relationship with this child and the relationship I had five years ago with my son, after I had given birth to him 'without knowing it'. The feeling of the passage of the baby from my own body into the world is absolutely unforgettable. It took me months to love my son, whereas the feeling which binds me to my daughter, who has just been born, is already extraordinarily strong, and I *know* that it is because I gave birth to her consciously. This is why, although I suffered during this confinement, I regard it as a success.

Mme R. Age: 31. Para. 2. 13 January, 1955. Boy 8 lb 6 oz

The father is urged to be present at his child's birth instead of being turned out, as is so often done in ordinary confinements. I did not agree with this previously. I would not have dared to prevent my husband from staying, but it would have disturbed me.

But now I am thrilled that he stayed with me until the end, and I shall never forget the moment when our son had just come out and was put on me. My husband came to kiss me, crying—because he was really crying. I was very moved. And even if the method had brought me only this joy, I should not regret having used it.

For any future labour, I would begin the same training again. Perhaps I shall have more luck, and everything will go well.

Opinion of a father. Sent by Dr. Monjardino of Lisbon

I have no medical knowledge, and my report has no scientific pretensions. My opinion is based on a personal experience which I felt intensely.

Our children were born in different countries. They were born under the care of well-known doctors and according to the most fashionable method of the time and place. I do not wish to criticize nor to flatter. Neither do I seek to make comparisons.

American method, 1941

For an American maternity clinic worthy of the name, the woman in labour is a patient, the child a most fragile being and the father a dangerous carrier of microbes.

The whole operation follows a plan. It is quite normal, after the official recognition of the pregnancy, to have to sign a contract with the gynaecologist—as we did—arranging his various services, before, during and after the confinement, those of his assistants, and the clinic, etc. An estimate is made and the whole is signed to make it valid. This satisfies practical minds. The family budget can be fixed, and the father-to-be is reassured about the care which his wife will receive. I doubt, however, if this reassures the mother-to-be to the same extent. She realizes too clearly what may happen to her.

Although she feels she is looked after with the greatest care, she regards her delivery as a sort of battle, and a battle is never joined without pain or blood. Although she is assured of all the material factors for victory, although a lot of preparations are made, especially when she goes to the clinic, the 'morale of the soldiers' is completely forgotten.

My wife was particularly courageous, and arrived at the clinic with a smile, but she was seized with panic before this mystery of life, and was made more panic-stricken by a great show of technique. What happened in the New York clinic, I do not know. When the husband has signed a good many papers and put his wife in the hands of the nurse on duty, he becomes a completely undesirable person, a real pariah full of bacteria that must be kept in a waiting-room.

I discussed this performance in the American hospital with many friends. Their reactions were all the same. Completely ignorant of what is happening to his wife, the husband is at first full of confident bravado. Time passes slowly, and he starts to read magazines dealing in detail with subjects as comforting as Caesarian operations or eclampsia—if it is not dyspepsia or infantile meningitis. In some hospitals, he is invited to a film performance dealing with the care of new-born babies and the subtle art of changing nappies.

When his supply of cigarettes is almost exhausted, and when he has worn out a few square yards of carpet, despair gives him the strength to venture into a corridor from which he is immediately repelled by the cold competent look of a nurse coming out of an autoclave.

And when he is completely crazy, at last the warm smile of the doctor appears bringing the good news and his congratulations. The husband's face is covered with a gauze mask, and he is admitted to the room where his wife recovers slowly from the anaesthetic.

The mother's first words are, 'It hurts.' Yet everything has happened normally. Her second words are: 'Have you seen the baby? Is he beautiful?' And then the father realizes that his wife has not even seen her child.

But where is the baby? The father has not seen him either.

He is in the aseptic day nursery, whimpering among other bundles just as anonymous. They are identified from a distance by a number, by looking through a port-hole of sealed glass. One cannot, of course, get near him under any pretext. Not even, as in my case, when one is at war, when one is an officer with marching orders, and one does not know if one will ever see him again.

This method is excellent with regard to the physical care of mother and baby. Nothing is forgotten; everything has been done. Science has given its best. But the mother remembers pain and discomfort, like a bad dream from which she is happy to wake. The father feels deeply humiliated. He is sorry that his wife went through this hard experience because of him. He swears not to do it again. Fortunately, the joys of motherhood make the mother forget her suffering, and all-powerful nature quickly makes a mock of the father's resolutions.

Method used in Belgium in 1947

The prenatal period proceeds with the necessary precautions almost as it would with the American method. However, there is no pre-established plan nor estimate.

The emphasis is placed on woman's rôle of reproduction. The duty of having children and the natural functions are insisted upon, which gives procreation a certain animal character. The aim is clearly to persuade the mother-to-be that there is no magic in what she does, that it is a normal act 'like digestion'. But all the same this removes the beauty of the act.

I believe that, unless the mother is a primitive being, her morale must be kept up by an appeal to higher feelings—the pride of creating life, the joy of a bigger family, the beauty of the mother-wife. It is usual to say to a woman: 'One must suffer to be beautiful' and so make her accept the inconveniences of fashion. One could just as well say to her: 'You must suffer a little to be a mother,' and obtain the same results.

At the time of confinement the mother is given an I/V injection of barbiturate, and the rest of the event occurs 'as though in a glass-house'. Everybody can see what is happening. The husband, of course, is also invited, but usually when the placenta is delivered—the least elegant moment in the story. He is thus face to face with a wife three-quarters unconscious and wandering, and a pile of blood-stained material which the doctor indifferently drops into a bowl. Animalism has been respected.

It seems that the barbiturate injection removes the most acute sensations of pain. Nevertheless, my wife, in her subconscious perhaps, must have felt these pains because she remembers them.

The baby is put near the mother, and she can see it as soon as she comes round. These injections have caused a very prolonged sleep and in our case they delayed lactation. Artificial stupor handicaps the realization that delivery is achieved. Consequently, the mother cannot feel any joy, the triumph which more than anything else makes her forget the trials of labour.

The father has naturally been much closer to events, and has been able to follow part of them. He is therefore under less strain, his paternal instinct has been more quickly touched and his responsibility has not been ignored. Nevertheless, even if he has strong nerves, he cannot prevent himself from feeling slightly disgusted. After all, he was only shown the miseries of birth, inevitable certainly, but too crudely revealed.

Later, his intimate life will be affected by it for a time. His wife too will feel a certain uneasiness.

Method used in Portugal in 1954 (by Dr. P. Monjardino)
When my wife came back from her doctor, and told me that he advocated a new method of childbirth requiring attendance at lectures and training in special breathing exercises, I was doubtful.

I thought—in spite of the respect and friendship that I have for our doctor—that it consisted of an experiment like the Coué method, or an attempt at hypnotism.

Then I found out more, and became convinced that this method was perfectly natural. I strongly advised my wife to follow the doctor's

suggestion and I encouraged her as much as I could. I am very glad
I made this decision.

Preparatory study: I consider this excellent, as much from the psychological as the practical point of view. Although my wife was already
well-informed on the subject—which must not always be so—she was
unaware of many details and some very interesting points. She took
notes and revised her lectures.

The lessons were clear, simple and detailed. They disregarded all
complications or accidents, so as to show the event in its most normal
light. This is very important. If the woman can be a help in a normal
confinement, what is the good of frightening her in advance by telling
her about extreme cases, when, anyway, only the intervention of the
man of science can save her?

These preparatory lectures create calmness and confidence. After
all, a chauffeur must know his car and how it works if he wants to drive
well. A woman, conscious and knowing about her functions, must feel
much more at ease and can, up to a certain point, direct her reactions.

I had two proofs of this. Contrary to the usual practice, my wife
did not tell me her last wishes just before the event, and did not dream
that anything could go wrong. Then, when she felt the first contractions, instead of the usual hurry and panic to leave for the clinic, she
said, very simply: 'The first protection has come away. We had better
get ready.'

And we left by car, driving slowly, joking and talking of the baby
as if he were born already.

The confinement: The first part of labour progressed much more
rapidly and with infinitely less pain than usual. The woman no longer
has 'pains' but 'contractions', which is indeed psychologically a good
substitute. My wife did not have that look of pain—nostrils narrowed,
eyes dilated and lips twisted. Her face was relaxed, almost smiling, and,
meanwhile, she was talking to me normally.

Twice she even doubted that the contractions were real; they were
so faint. And we had to confirm that the cervix was dilating to convince her. The quick respiration is certainly the cause of the satisfactory
state—and also the use of oxygen. The quick respiration took her mind
off the event by giving her something to do. It is certain that this way of
breathing has other effects of relaxation and maintaining strength.

Even during the war, we were advised to breathe quickly and
irregularly when we had to make special physical efforts or when we
were under fire. The aim and the results must be the same in labour,

I would say, however, that, since each person breathes in her own way, it is difficult to teach this breathing along general lines. But the doctor should study and define the respiration of the woman, or else she should train herself much longer. The benefits of quick respiration lessen after more than an hour, on account of the tiredness which it causes when the contractions are very close together. This fatigue could be delayed or decreased if the woman adapted her respiration.

Oxygen has an extraordinary effect, and my wife, who never tires of praising it, felt all the better for it, not only during labour which was made so much easier, but also after labour when she felt stronger.

There were other important details, including the foam-rubber mattress, which gives a pleasant foundation and prevents pains in the back and even the bruises that one used to get on hard tables.

Now I must describe my impressions again.

This time, I was invited by the doctor to be present at the confinement and even to take a modest part in it. I gave the oxygen. I was glad of this for I did not feel excluded from an important moment of my married life, nor humiliated nor disgusted. I was able to follow step by step the progress of events, and, as these were well prepared and my wife in good form, I found the operation interesting. There was no need for me to get restive since I saw what was happening. I had a job to do, and felt a duty and responsibility which banished any sordidness.

My wife assures me that my presence was a help and comfort to her, especially at the time of delivery. This last part seemed to me like the 'finale' of a symphony. At a certain moment, the doctor took command, and my wife began to obey him instinctively. Seated beside her, I pressed her hand at each effort, and then put the oxygen mask, flowing at three litres a minute, on her face. It seemed as though the doctor's voice, the will-power (and perhaps the strength) that I communicated to my wife and the co-ordinated efforts of a willing, controlled push, blended into one unique action which resulted in the birth.

It was an extraordinary sensation to see my son appear and feel that I was his father at his first cry.   And later on, when my wife was in her room and we looked at the cradle with some emotion, we told each other: 'We made this baby together, from the beginning to the end.'

This feeling of union and community is of great importance. It gives the woman a feeling of pure joy which immediately brings her energy, the more so as her previous achievement in overcoming the pain has left her in a state of euphoria and able to recover quickly. I myself felt just simply happy.

I congratulate the doctors on having discovered a natural method of childbirth without pain and thank our doctor for the masterly way in which he succeeded. This method is within the capacity of everyone. All women, rich or poor, can obtain the same results. Only good willpower and training are needed. Women will also learn a little more, which in itself is something.

In conclusion we would urge that every possible means should be used to bring recognition to C.W.P. It should be used in hospitals and maternity centres, and should not be allowed to fall into disrepute through misapplication or malicious abuse.

We believe we have proved its value. Facilities should now be provided for all children to come into the world in joy, for the happiness of their parents and the benefit of society.

Conclusion

I T is the woman who gives birth. But without the psychoprophylactic method, she would still be kept out of the picture. In the past, giving birth implied inactivity; as if the events that she experienced within herself during pregnancy and childbirth were in some way imposed upon her from without and followed an almost mysterious course. The stages became apparent to her only through the jargon of the doctors. And even when it was not very painful, labour subdued the woman, who was already inhibited by ignorance which had been carefully cultivated during the nine months. And it confined her in a vegetative world. Today, childbirth has become an active phenomenon. Through it woman can completely find herself and express herself as a human being.

To say 'It is the woman who gives birth' also emphasizes the dynamic character of the method. It really requires the opinion of women, not only for it to become more and more effective, but for it simply to come into being in the first place. Psychoprophylaxis involves discussion and exchange of ideas.

Over the last five years, the method has made considerable progress. It has been submitted to constant criticism, which is becoming more rigorous now that many women are experiencing their second childbirth without pain. It has met with success, but also with failure, the causes of which have often been analysed by the women themselves. There is an increasing demand for the method as results improve.

It has taken root. The lectures have become more detailed and complete. Certain ideas have dropped out, because they seemed too elementary. Women have gradually realized the situation through increasing use of the method and various articles written about it. The aim proposed by Velvoski in Russia, 'suppression of pain in labour considered as an established and widespread social phenomenon,' has begun to be achieved in France. Women are better equipped and informed and want a higher level of education. The psychoprophylactic method can hope to come into general use. Certainly, in the last four years, it has spread all over France, and from France crossed many

frontiers. Not all obstetricians have adopted it yet. Although the number of critics and opponents has considerably diminished, some remain.
What is more, we cannot be sure that all those who have adopted it
use it *as it should be used*. There are many pseudo-converts, and in
various ways they distort it because in certain respects it inconveniences
them. They also put down to the method failures for which they are
responsible.

But opposition really arises because childbirth without pain brings
into question all the ideas and attitudes of the past—the inevitable
character of the pain, the passive rôle of the woman.

A specialist, whose interest in the psychoprophylactic method
was undoubted, once made this heart-breakingly obvious remark:
'I have discovered that it is necessary to study childbirth alongside
the woman in the labour ward in order to understand the principles of the method and to perfect our own attitude to it.' Yes,
indeed.

But what does it matter? What is important is that the social
phenomenon has been established. The arguments which were bound
to occur during the first phases of the struggle may now be forgotten.
No one can deny that childbirth without pain has taken place. It
exists, will develop, and transform the lives of more and more women
each day. The late Pope, in his discourse of 8 January, 1956, not only
recognized its existence but gave it his moral approval. This is a
development of great importance, because, in lifting the ban which
many Catholics had cast over a materialistic method, he gave it a
chance of penetrating into new layers of society. At the same time, he
put women in a position to reject false methods.

'To know more, better, and sooner,' a profound desire. The
teaching has liberated childbirth and pregnancy from the taboos with
which tradition surrounded them. It has encouraged women to understand the mystery, to visualize the invisible. It has pushed back the
frontiers of maternity, in making the mother familiar with the various
manifestations of life in the uterus.

The lectures now start as early as possible. It was all right to say
to the women: 'This is what happened inside you from the beginning
of your pregnancy.' But it is far better to say, 'This is what is happening.' Knowledge of the events as they appear is one of the best means
of avoiding the troubles which often accompany them. Practical
exercises are added to the teaching to influence the organic and functional changes of pregnancy. But the most important advantage is

that the positive physiological effect of words can be exerted for a longer time and more profoundly.

The unity of the method

The method is constantly confronted with new facts, but the principle of its teaching remains permanent and unchangeable. Physiology is neither cortical nor visceral; it is cortico-visceral. Pavlov's comment was emphasized in the last lecture. And we can never insist upon this too much. Theory and practice are inseparable; and, as we have seen, so are the mind and the body, and, in the same way, the various elements in the training. The woman learns the structure of the internal organs, especially the uterus; she realizes the function of each of these organs, as well as the mechanical and chemical changes that pregnancy and childbirth create in them. She must not forget that her physical exercises affect both the organ concerned and her *brain*, the sensory threshold of which they raise. Inversely, mental deconditioning, combined with knowledge, has a direct influence on the quality of the organ's function. Neuromuscular training assumes its full meaning only if it is accompanied by training in respiration, and both of them together have their full effect only if they are related to an understanding of the theory.

The psychoprophylactic method strictly follows the principles of the science from which it is derived. While the brain—which analyses, synthesizes and controls—unifies the body, the body affects the brain. It modifies the brain's activity as a result of changes in itself. Cortico-visceral physiology, in describing the interdependent systems which make up the human body, shows that man is a whole. Each of his parts is inseparable from the others. To be painless, childbirth must obey this fundamental rule, and must not exclude—or not favour at the expense of others—any part of this complex whole which constitutes a woman in labour.

Certain errors or risks of error must be mentioned. Except in pathological cases, the success of childbirth and the good progress of pregnancy are dependent upon the good functioning of the brain. But this could never mean that the brain alone is responsible, that the brain controls everything. It had, as it were, to be revived. Its tone had to be restored. It had to become able again to analyse, synthesize, control and co-ordinate. It had to be freed from inhibition caused by ignorance. But the fact that the brain thus recovered, through a rational education, a sensory threshold able to stop the sensations coming from the uterus, does not remove all risk. A contraction, if it is hampered by any organic factor, may become a signal of pain. It is necessary to keep constant watch—and the brain plays an important part here in keeping the woman alert—on the physiological harmony of the various phases of childbirth; not to cause any obstacle to it; to carry out all the activities of response that it demands. When the woman does the breathing badly, she suffers, and she stops suffering as soon as she does it well.

Although the woman must become capable, by a deeper awareness, of dissociating various types of muscular actions, the dissociation is only a stage in the working out of the method. It reveals one aspect of the situation and not the situation itself. Errors of interpretation have been made. To help understand one of the essential mechanisms of the brain, its 'braking power', the example used to be given of a traveller wearied by the noise of train and conversations. He buries himself in a book, manages to ignore the noise and isolates himself completely. Another example is the soldier who for a time ignores his wound because the battle absorbs all his attention.

These examples carry a danger. It may be thought that a woman can be distracted from childbirth by work to which she gives all her attention. In childbirth ᵗhe situation is different. The traveller is not aware of the train; he ignores it and does not worry about the way it is running. The soldier is not aware of his wound; he does not know where it is, how serious it is, nor what should be done for it. On the other hand, the woman becomes completely aware of her body and of the different stages of childbirth. She is especially aware of the contraction, the essential event of childbirth. She has learned what she must do, and her work responds exactly. It does not distract her; does not divert her from her situation. It is adaptation, *integration*.

The idea of will-power is also very dangerous. If the woman has not learned what is happening, nor what she must do at such and such a moment, no will-power will make up for this lack, will make her brain capable of stopping all the sensations coming from her body in labour. And her will-power must especially not be used to try to isolate her from childbirth, since this requires her whole active presence.

The practical exercises, which the women are taught, are closely related to theory, as well as to the various organic changes in pregnancy and childbirth. They cannot be regarded as simple 'gymnastics', whether they are considered as essential or secondary. These exercises must be *directed* and *controlled* carefully. They are somewhat briefly described in the preceding pages but *none of them should be done without medical direction.*

We must mention one more development. One day a woman complained of her relations' doubt and mockery about the method—especially the film which concludes the lectures and in which they see a confinement. 'We know what films are,' the mother said sceptically to her daughter. 'We know that they're faked.'

The young woman, although a very good pupil, was adversely influenced by this attitude, which was bound to upset her deconditioning. There was only one thing to do—direct teaching. The young woman, with several of her companions, watched an actual confinement. The experiment was, of course, completely conclusive, and her first reaction was to run to her mother and tell her 'I have *seen* a confinement!'

In present conditions this experiment cannot, unfortunately, become the general rule; but while we wait for things to improve, it will be repeated as often as possible. Maternity, in its very reality, must be part of education and not be excluded from it as if it were a terrible mystery or a shameful event.

The husband was not mentioned in the past, except perhaps in enquiries about his job and health insurance number. He was tolerated in certain clinics only on condition that he kept out of the way. Now his existence and individuality are recognized. He becomes the husband and the father again. He was often mentioned when the psychoprophylactic method began; and gradually he was more and more required to help his wife revise the lectures, keep an eye on her practical exercises, and if necessary support her during her confinement. But he was approached through his wife, and this amounted in fact to his being kept in the background. Today, his presence and his active collaboration are sought. Thus the couple are no longer separated. It is the couple from now on that we address.

A method such as this should be made available to all couples. It should be used in all maternity homes. But it is upon women that the early achievement of a programme of this sort depends. Although ten, fifteen, a hundred people who have experienced it may insist in articles or speeches that the psychoprophylactic method must be applied, their influence cannot be compared with the pressure which women themselves can bring to bear. It is up to those who use the maternity homes to demand the method. They have already exerted pressure to improve the method itself—thus necessitating the publication of this book. As long as they know how to ask for it, they will get what they want. No one can oppose those who are experienced, educated and well-informed—and know what they want.

Childbirth, which has been entirely under the Ministry of Health, should in future come under the Ministry of Education. Maternity, the social phenomenon, must be studied at school. To win this second battle, Dr. Lamaze relied in the first place on women.